Food exchanges for over 3,000

supermarket, grocery store,

and fast-food products.

Compiled and written by
Andrea Barrett

With a foreword by
Charles R. Shuman, M.D.

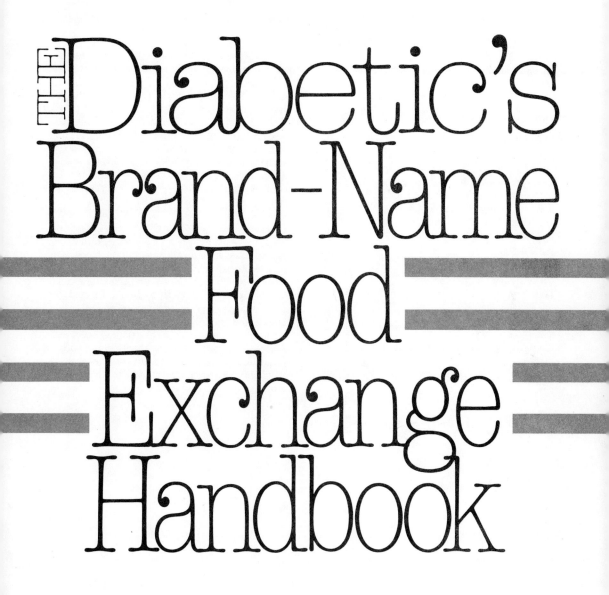

The Diabetic's Brand-Name Food Exchange Handbook

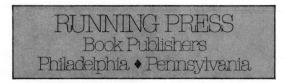

RUNNING PRESS
Book Publishers
Philadelphia ◆ Pennsylvania

9   8   7   6   5   4   3   2   1
The digit on the right indicates the number of this printing.

Library of Congress Cataloging in Publication Data: Barrett, Andrea.   The diabetic's brand-name food exchange handbook.   Includes index.
1. Diabetes—Diet therapy. 2. Food—Tables.
3. Brand name products. I. Title. [DNLM:
1. Diabetic diet—Handbooks. WK 819 B274d]
RC662.B34 1984   616.4'620654   84–2105
ISBN 0-89471-256-X
ISBN 0-89471-237-3 (lib. bdg.)

Cover design by Toby Schmidt. Typography: Paladium, American Typewriter, and Helios by rci, Philadelphia, PA. Printed by Port City Press, Baltimore, MD.

This book may be ordered by mail from the publisher. Please include 95 cents postage. *But try your bookstore first.* Running Press Book Publishers, 125 South 22nd Street, Philadelphia, Pennsylvania 19103.

ACKNOWLEDGMENTS

My thanks to the many food manufacturers who graciously provided nutrient values from which exchanges were calculated. Best, Burger King, Campbell's, Calco, Dairy Queen/Brazier, Dia-Mel, Estee, Hardee's, Heinz, Hormel, Kellogg's, Kentucky Fried Chicken, Louis Rich, McDonald's, Nabisco, Oscar Mayer, Pillsbury, Stouffer's, Swift, Weight Watchers, and Worthington companies provided exchanges as well as nutrient values, which were adapted as necessary. They deserve special thanks for their efforts to make prepared products accessible to diabetics.

Judith Wylie–Rosett, Ed.D., R.D., Assistant Professor, Departments of Community Health and Medicine, Albert Einstein College of Medicine, provided the exchanges for Heinz baby foods and reviewed Chapter 10. Barbara Herbst, M.S., R.D., Chief Research Dietitian, General Clinical Research Center, Temple University Hospital, calculated all other exchanges, provided invaluable nutritional advice, and critically reviewed the manuscript. Charles R. Shuman, M.D., Professor of Medicine, Temple University School of Medicine, provided the foreword and sound medical advice. This book would not have been possible without their hard work, support, and guidance.

Foreword

DIABETES—AN OVERVIEW

Diabetes affects nearly 11 million people in the United States alone. In recent years, new knowledge of its causes has emerged, demonstrating clearly that diabetes is not a single disease, but rather a group of conditions associated with *hyperglycemia* (elevated blood sugar).

Elevated blood sugar may result if the pancreas does not secrete enough insulin. Some diabetics, however, have what we call *insulin resistance*. They have an insulin response similar to that of non-diabetics, but are unable to use the insulin they secrete to lower their blood sugar levels. Obesity is associated with insulin resistance, and overweight diabetics may continue to secrete large amounts of insulin even though their fasting blood sugar levels are high. It is important to realize that the pancreas's ability to produce insulin can be exhausted by this combination of long-standing obesity and hyperglycemia. In response to a rise in blood sugar, less insulin is secreted than is required; the result may be insulin dependence. Conversely, weight reduction can often reverse insulin resistance.

In 1979, the National Diabetes Data Group, an international work group sponsored by the National Institutes of Health, developed a practical classification of diabetes mellitus and other categories of glucose intolerance. Diabetes was subdivided into three different types, based primarily on the underlying causes of the disease.

Type I—insulin-dependent diabetes mellitus (IDDM)—affects

approximately 15% of all diabetics. These people have lost most or all of their insulin-secreting tissue (the pancreatic islets) due to damage by viral infection or by antibodies which react with these tissues. Typically, they have a rapid onset of symptoms which may progress to diabetic ketoacidosis (DKA) if not recognized and treated with insulin. Type I diabetes is related to genetic factors involving the immune system. It occurs most often in young people, but may occur at any age.

Type II—non-insulin-dependent diabetes (NIDDM)—occurs in 80% of the diabetic population, and has a genetic basis unrelated to the immune system. Seen most frequently in adults, it may also occur in young members of families affected by this type of diabetes. Obesity is an important factor, affecting 60% to 90% of these patients. Excessive caloric intake, resulting in weight gain, leads to persistent hyperglycemia; weight loss improves the condition. In Type II diabetics, insulin deficiency is less striking, while insulin resistance is more important as a cause of abnormal blood sugar concentrations. Type II diabetics may have few or no symptoms for many years, but under stress or during infection they may develop the more severe manifestations observed in Type I diabetics.

Other Types—secondary diabetes—occur rarely, in association with certain endocrine disorders, following disease involving the pancreas, or with a variety of genetic syndromes.

Efforts to improve the treatment of diabetes have given both patients and physicians new and effective methods for blood sugar control. One important innovation has been home blood-glucose monitoring, which enables diabetics to adjust their insulin doses and dietary intake for the most effective regulation of blood sugar levels.

Crucial in the management of diabetes is an understanding of its nutritional aspects. Diet therapy can help prevent or delay the cardiovascular, renal, retinal, and neurological complications of diabetes. The Committee on Nutrition of the American Diabetes Association advocates a balanced intake of carbohydrate, fat, and protein food sources in meal planning. The Committee recommends regular, uniform meals to ensure a consistent availability of the nutritional elements required to maintain normal function of all tissues. A diabetic's diet should be designed to accommodate the individual's eating habits, with appropriate modifications to satisfy nutritional needs and avoid excessive amounts of refined sugars and saturated fats.

Traditional dietary management of diabetes is based on the arrangement of foods into groups. In 1950, the American Diabetes Association, The American Dietetic Association, and the U.S. Public Health Service devised the *Food Exchange System*, using six lists of food. This system permits the selection of a wide variety of foods, each of equivalent caloric value, from the specific lists. Portions are determined by household measurements. Diets are individualized for each patient, who receives careful instruction and counseling from a physician, dietitian, and diabetes teaching nurse so as to select the proper foods for his or her daily schedule.

Using this system, the total caloric intake and the distribution of food can be kept reasonably consistent with minimum regimentation, while preserving eating pleasure. This book has been prepared with these important objectives in mind.

Charles R. Shuman, M.D.
Professor of Medicine
Temple University School of Medicine

TABLE OF CONTENTS

HOW—AND WHEN—
TO USE THIS BOOK

This book contains information you won't find anywhere else. It's not just a listing of nutrient values or calories, but *new* information to help make living with diabetes easier. You can use this book to help understand nutrition labels on prepared foods in your supermarket, to choose foods both tasty and good for you, and to design exciting and varied meals that fit into your prescribed meal plan. You can also refer to it when you're eating at a friend's house or a fast-food restaurant and you want to fit "complicated" foods into your meal plan.

Most of all, this book helps you work within the limits of your calorie-controlled exchange diet, often referred to as the "ADA Diet" because it's based on information contained in *Exchange Lists for Meal Planning*, a booklet developed in 1950 and revised in 1976 by committees of the American Diabetes Association and The American Dietetic Association. (If you don't already have a copy, you can get one from either of these associations or their affiliate organizations.) If you're an insulin-dependent (Type I) diabetic, a version of this diet prepared by your physician or dietitian will help you maintain appropriate blood sugar levels, avoiding prolonged periods of hyperglycemia as well as potentially dangerous insulin reactions. If you're an overweight, non-insulin-dependent (Type II) diabetic, this diet will help you lose weight (the single most effective way of controlling diabetes) while keeping your blood sugar within normal limits. If you're not diabetic, but are simply overweight, this diet (recommended by many physicians for simple weight loss) is safe, effective, and well-balanced in terms of carbohydrate, protein, and fat. It can help you restrict calories without a loss of important nutrients.

In the exchange system, foods are grouped into the six "Exchange Lists" shown below:*

EXCHANGE LIST	GRAMS OF CARBOHYDRATE	GRAMS OF PROTEIN	GRAMS OF FAT	CALORIES
Fat	0	0	5	45
Milk	12	8	0	80
Vegetable	5	2	0	25[1]
Fruit	10	0	0	40
Bread	15	2	0	70[2]
Meat:				
Lean	0	7	3	55
Medium-fat	0	7	5	75[3]
High-fat	0	7	8	100

Based on these exchange lists, your dietitian will design a specific diet for you, balanced in terms of the number of calories derived from protein, carbohydrate, and fat. Depending on the number of calories you need, you'll be allowed a certain number of exchanges from each group for every meal and snack. Foods within a list contain similar amounts of calories, protein, carbohydrate, and fat, and may be freely exchanged with all other foods in that list. You'll find, for instance, that one slice of rye bread is equal to half a hamburger bun or half a cup of cooked rice, or that one ounce of lean beef is equal to a quarter-cup of 2% cottage cheese or the same amount of canned tuna.

The *Exchange Lists for Meal Planning* includes many basic, unprocessed foods, such as vegetables, fruits, breads, and meats. Other lists, such as the *Expanded Guide to Meal Planning* (Illinois Nutrition Educators, Inc., 1979) and the supplementary lists in *The American Diabetes Association/The American Dietetic Association Family Cookbook* (Prentice-Hall, 1980) include additional items such as ethnic foods and specialty vegetables.

But it's tough to stay on a regimented diet day after day, and these exchange lists don't include brand-name *prepared* foods—all those frozen, canned, jarred, preserved, dried, and baked items that line supermarket shelves and fill vending machines, tempting you with their

---

*The exchange lists are based on material in *Exchange Lists for Meal Planning*, prepared by committees of the American Diabetes Association, Inc., and The American Dietetic Association, in cooperation with the National Institute of Arthritis, Metabolism and Digestive Diseases and the National Heart and Lung Institute, National Institutes of Health, Public Health Service, U.S. Department of Health, Education, and Welfare. Reprinted with permission.

[1] Actual value is 28. Rounded-off figures are used for convenience.
[2] Actual value is 68.
[3] Actual value is 73.

convenience and variety. You don't have to avoid them, just because they aren't listed in your exchange lists. The American Diabetes Association's "Special Report: Principles of Nutrition and Dietary Recommendations for Individuals with Diabetes Mellitus" (1979) recommends allowing "the widest possible options in food choices and distribution of food intake . . . consistent with fundamentals of good nutrition and the approval of the attending physician."* Your physician and dietitian know that the variety of prepared foods can make staying on your diet easier, without jeopardizing good nutrition.

And that's where this book comes in. When you want to enjoy the convenience of Green Giant Lasagna with Meat Sauce for dinner, *that's* when you use this book. Here, you'll find thousands of brand-name foods listed with their caloric content and their exchanges already calculated. For instance, one serving of Green Giant Lasagna with Meat Sauce contains 470 calories, 2½ bread exchanges, 2 meat exchanges, 1 vegetable exchange, and 3½ fat exchanges. Knowing this, you can then easily see how (or sometimes, unfortunately, *whether*) that lasagna fits into your meal plan.

As for *how* to use this book, you'll find brand-name foods arranged by category here, rather than in strict alphabetical order. For instance, all frozen lasagna dishes are grouped together in Chapter 1, under the heading **COMBINATION MAIN DISHES—Frozen**. Calories and exchanges are *not* always the same in similar products made by different manufacturers, so if you're making a shopping list, you'll be able to consider similar foods, see how each fits into your meal plan, and compare different brands of the same item.

Notice that items which include meat exchanges are not divided into lean, medium-fat, and high-fat categories. Since medium-fat and high-fat meat exchanges are really nothing but lean meat exchanges plus fat, *all* products in this book were calculated in terms of lean meat exchanges plus fat exchanges. Again, the idea is for you to be able to compare products more easily.

If you're used to working with medium-fat and high-fat meat exchanges, some foods listed here will seem to have a large number of fat exchanges—sometimes too many to fit into your meal plan. Look closely at the exchanges you're allowed for a given meal. If a particular product exceeds your allowed number of fat exchanges for that meal, but you have medium-fat or high-fat meat exchanges available, you can convert the exchanges as follows:

1 medium-fat exchange	equals	1 lean meat exchange
	plus	½ fat exchange
1 high-fat meat exchange	equals	1 lean meat exchange
	plus	1 fat exchange

---

*Diabetes Care 2(6):520

As you can see, one ounce of cheddar cheese equals 1 high-fat meat exchange *or* 1 lean meat exchange plus 1 fat exchange. Similarly, the 3 medium-fat meat exchanges you might be allowed at dinner are also equal to 3 lean meat exchanges plus 1½ fat exchanges.

In addition to giving the exchanges for each item, we've also included the number of calories per serving—as reported by the manufacturer. Exchanges are seldom exact; if you compare the calories listed with those you get by adding up the exchanges, you'll often find a small difference. However, if you eat a variety of foods, the differences tend to even out.

Serving sizes are those listed as given by the manufacturer. If you pick up a can of Armour Chili without Beans (15 ounces) and see that the serving size listed is 7½ ounces (½ can), that's how you'll find the product listed in this book.

You'll also notice that some serving sizes are expressed as whole numbers and others as fractions or decimal numbers. We've left the suggested serving sizes exactly as they appear on the package labels to save you the trouble of converting from one form to another.

If you plan to eat more or less than the amount given as the serving size, adjust exchanges accordingly. As with any measured diet, be careful about portions. If you've worked 10 Rich and Crisp crackers (1½ bread exchanges plus 1 fat exchange) into your meal plan, don't eat 14 of them! Many serving sizes are listed in ounces, so you'll want to keep your food scale handy. However, you'll find that some of these foods also list the number of servings per package on the label, which allows you to arrive at the correct portion size by dividing the package contents by the number of servings. A 15-ounce can of chili, for instance, might list the serving size as 5 ounces and the number of servings per can as three. Using exactly one-third of the can will give you the correct portion without weighing.

Some prepared foods, particularly mixes, require you to add certain ingredients. Wherever possible, exchanges are given for these products *as prepared according to package directions.* If a boxed macaroni and cheese mix calls for the addition of whole milk and butter, then exchanges will be calculated using these ingredients. If you make substitutions, like using skim milk instead of whole milk, adjust the exchanges accordingly. When directions offer a choice of ingredients (such as adding milk *or* water to a condensed soup), we've indicated which ingredient was used for the exchange calculation.

Certain foods are listed here as "free," others as "free in moderation." The difference is important. "Free" foods, those with no sugar and few or no calories, do not affect your blood sugar, and won't cause you to gain weight. Therefore, you may eat them whenever you want. There's a supplementary list of free foods at the end of this book (Appendix II), so that you can find them all at a glance. Foods shown as "free in moderation" are foods that, *in the serving size listed*, have less than 20 calories and don't have to be counted as an exchange. But they do have *some* calories, and those calories can add up. While 1 tablespoon of A-1 Steak Sauce (12 calories) can be used "freely" with your dinner, 5 tablespoons would add up to 60 calories—almost as much as a bread exchange. "Free in moderation" means just that. Use these items to add spice to your diet—but use them in the amounts suggested. Appendix II also lists free-in-moderation foods.

Finally, you'll find a few sugar-sweetened cakes and cookies listed in Chapter 5. These items, marked with (*) for your convenience, should be used only occasionally and only with your physician's approval. Insulin-dependent diabetics who use home blood-glucose monitoring systems may want to use these items during vigorous short-term physical activity. These foods are also useful in preventing insulin reactions. The exchanges are listed here because, on the rare occasions when you do eat these foods, you'll want to be able to figure them into your meal plan.

In Appendix III, you'll find some additional sugar-sweetened foods useful for providing concentrated carbohydrate during sick days. Other than that, most sugar-sweetened foods aren't listed here. Instead, you'll find in Chapter 8 a long list of "sweets" containing aspartame (NutraSweet), fructose, saccharin, or sorbitol instead of sugar. If your sweet tooth isn't satisfied by a piece of fresh fruit, choose one of these items instead. Remember, though, that the label "dietetic" doesn't mean "diabetic" or "noncaloric." Foods sweetened with nutritive sweeteners sometimes contain as many calories as their sugar-sweetened counterparts—and they must be counted in your daily meal plan.

The chapter introductions give more specific information about each group of foods and how to use them in your meal plan. A table of measurements (Appendix I) will help you understand serving sizes and make conversions as needed. Agencies and organizations listed in Appendix IV can help you find a physician or dietitian, and can provide advice about your diet and all aspects of your diabetes. Appendix VI provides sample exchange patterns at different calorie levels. For the mathematically-minded, there's a section on "Calculating Exchanges for Other Brand-Name Foods" (Appendix V), which can help you with foods not listed here. You'll find that calculating exchanges really isn't difficult. Once you get the hang of it, you can work all sorts of new foods into your meal plan.

Sensible use of prepared foods in a meal plan based on exchange lists *can* be good for you. But this book is meant to be used with the advice and support of your physician and dietitian. Consult with them, and then enjoy yourself!

SOURCES OF PRODUCT INFORMATION

Serving sizes, calorie content, and carbohydrate, protein, and fat content were obtained directly from food manufacturers and are listed as provided.

Barbara Herbst, M.S., R.D., of the General Clinical Research Center of Temple University Hospital (Philadelphia, PA) calculated most exchanges from the nutritional data. Some exchanges were provided directly by the manufacturer (Best, Burger King, Campbell's, Calco, Dairy Queen/Brazier, Dia-Mel, Estee, Hardee's, Heinz, Hormel, Kellogg's, Kentucky Fried Chicken, Louis Rich, McDonald's, Nabisco, Oscar Mayer, Pillsbury,* Stouffer's, Swift, Weight Watchers, and Worthington companies), and then checked for accuracy and adapted as appropriate, according to the guidelines explained in the following section. All exchanges provided by food manufacturers were converted from high- and medium-fat meat exchanges to lean meat exchanges, as necessary.

Alcoholic beverage information was obtained from the Anheuser-Busch, Heublein, Miller, and Pabst companies, and from USDA Handbook #456, *Nutritive Value of American Foods in Common Units.*

Every effort has been made to obtain the most current and accurate data available. Product formulations *do* change, however, as do product sizes. Compare the labels of products you buy with the information listed

---

*The exchange values listed may differ from Pillsbury's published diabetic exchange lists, which were calculated in terms of high-fat and medium-fat meat exchanges.

in this book. If the serving sizes or calories listed for a particular item differ from those listed here, or if the product is described as "new" or "improved," ask your dietitian to check the exchanges—or check them yourself, using the steps in Appendix V.

You may find that some of your favorite foods aren't included. Many sugar-sweetened foods have been omitted because they're inappropriate for most diabetics. Other foods weren't included because their manufacturers didn't have the necessary information available, or were changing product formulations. Still other items are marketed on a strictly regional basis. To find the appropriate exchanges for these items, use Appendix V.

This book is designed to be a teaching guide as well as a reference manual. Nothing presented here is "special" in any way—the information used to calculate exchanges for this book is essentially the same information you'll find on product labels, except that figures on product labels are rounded off to the nearest whole number. If product labeling is unclear or incomplete, write the Consumer Service Department of the product's manufacturer. In most cases you'll find them prompt to respond and eager to help.

This book is meant to be used with the knowledge and support of your physician and dietitian. The information presented here is based on research and consultation with authorities in the fields of diabetes and nutrition. Every effort has been made to present the most accurate and current information, but since information was obtained from many sources, inaccuracies or inconsistencies may occur. The author and the publisher disclaim responsibility for any adverse effects resulting directly or indirectly from use of the information in this book.

A NOTE FOR PHYSICIANS, DIETITIANS, AND OTHERS PROVIDING DIET COUNSELING FOR DIABETICS

This book is designed to help you and your patients make the most effective use of exchange lists. As you design meal plans that promote good diabetes control and diet compliance, you may need to adjust exchanges to correspond to different serving sizes, or calculate new exchanges for foods not listed here. The following guidelines, used in this book for calculating exchanges, may be helpful to you:

•The actual values for bread and vegetable exchanges as derived from the grams of carbohydrate and protein (68 and 28 calories, respectively) have been used in calculations, rather than the rounded-off figures of 70 and 25 calories found in ADA exchange lists.

•All meat exchanges are for lean meat (7 grams protein, 3 grams fat, 55 calories), so that patients can easily compare the amount of fat found in different foods. When food manufacturers did not provide exchanges in this form, we converted them to lean meat exchanges plus fat as follows: one medium-fat meat exchange (7 grams protein, 5 grams fat, 73 calories) equals one lean meat exchange (55 calories) plus one-half fat exchange (22 calories). One high-fat meat exchange (7 grams protein, 8 grams fat, 100 calories) equals one lean meat exchange (55 calories) plus one fat exchange (45 calories). Although some poultry items and vegetarian meat substitutes have less fat than a lean meat exchange, we haven't used "negative" fat exchanges since many patients find them confusing. Many patients also find it difficult to deal with three meat subgroups, so you may want to provide them with a meal plan calculated in terms of lean meat exchanges plus fat. The *Diet Counselor's Supplement to Expanded Guide to Meal Planning* (1979; available from Illinois Nutrition Educators, Inc., Box 1386, Evanston, IL 60204) offers useful suggestions for integrating the three meat subgroups into meal plans.

•Exchanges are shown to the nearest half exchange (half an exchange is defined as half the number of grams, rounded off, of carbohydrate, protein, or fat, multiplied by 4, 4, or 9 calories per gram, respectively). Exchanges less than ¼ were dropped; those from ¼ to ¾ were counted as ½; those from ¾ to 1¼ were counted as 1; and so forth.

•For each item, we tried to make the caloric value reported by the manufacturer agree with both the caloric value of the item's exchanges and the caloric value calculated from its carbohydrate, protein, and fat content. In order to do this, several approximations were necessary:

—The total caloric value for each item calculated from exchanges differs from the manufacturer's reported caloric value by no more than 20 calories. If the manufacturer provided both exchanges and total calories, and the caloric value we derived from these exchanges differed from the caloric value by more than 20 calories, we modified the exchanges to be within 20 calories of the reported caloric value.

—If the calorie count reported by the manufacturer differed by more than 20 calories from that derived by multiplying the reported grams of carbohydrate, protein, and fat by the number of calories per gram, we didn't include the item. When this difference was less than 20 calories, we calculated exchanges so that their caloric value would fall between the derived and the reported values.

•So that label information and exchanges can be easily compared, serving sizes for most products are those reported by the manufacturer. We made a few exceptions when a common serving size was significantly different than the one reported. Bread, for instance, was calculated on a one-slice basis rather than the two slices often reported by manufacturers —since one slice is the basis for the ADA bread exchange. Some serving sizes were reduced for free-in-moderation foods, primarily condiments, to keep the calorie count under 20.

•We calculated exchanges on the basis of how well the product's ingredients reflected the nutrient content of that exchange group, as well as on the basis of calories and grams of carbohydrate, protein, and fat. Vegetable exchanges, for example, were not used for the catsup on a fast-food burger, nor was catsup alone considered a vegetable. Fruit exchanges were used only where actual fruit was present, and were not used to represent sugar content (except for fructose and sorbitol). Cereals such as raisin bran did not contain enough fruit to justify use of a fruit exchange. Nuts and nut butters are shown as fat exchanges plus meat exchanges and bread exchanges (used if the item contained more than 5 grams of carbohydrate per serving), reflecting their nutrient content. Bread exchanges which appear in items with no obvious bread items are used to account for cornstarch or other carbohydrate thickeners. When the manufacturer provided sugar content for dry, ready-to-eat cereals, we included only those with a sugar content less than 28% of the total carbohydrate content and less than 25% of the total calories for unfruited cereals, and less than 36% of the total carbohydrate content and less than 36% of the total calories for fruited cereals.

•Current research on the effects of various complex carbohydrates and simple sugars (particularly sucrose) on blood sugar levels may offer new ways of working these foods into meal plans, but a complete index of glycemic responses to carbohydrates is not yet available.* Lacking this, we have grouped the complex carbohydrate foods into a bread exchange, as is traditionally done. However, anticipating that health-care professionals may in the future allow a modest amount of sucrose in the diabetic meal plan, we have included some cookies and cakes (not iced or filled with sweet creams or frostings) in Chapter 5. Although we couldn't determine the percentage of sugar in these items, cakes and cake mixes with more than 35 grams of carbohydrate per serving and cookies with more than 20 grams of carbohydrate per serving were not included. The carbohydrate in these items has been calculated as bread exchanges. Relatively few cakes and cookies are listed here, but the presence of any particular item does not imply an endorsement.

---

*See Bantle, J.P., *et al.*, *New Engl. J. Med.* 309:7, 1983, and *Science*, 220:487, 1983. For a partial index of glycemic responses, see Jenkins, D.J.A., *et al.*, *Am. J. Clin. Nutr.* 34:362, 1981.

ABBREVIATIONS

EXCHANGES

B	bread exchange	V	vegetable exchange
M	lean meat exchange	Fr	fruit exchange
F	fat exchange	Mk	nonfat milk exchange

MEASUREMENTS

fl. oz.	fluid ounce (volume)	tbsp.	tablespoon
lb.	pound	tsp.	teaspoon
oz.	ounce (weight)	g	gram
pkg.	package	cals	kilocalories
pt.	pint	mg	milligram
qt.	quart	ml	milliliter

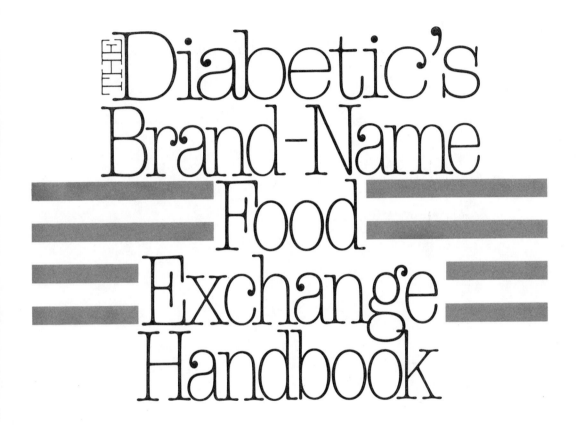

THE Diabetic's Brand-Name Food Exchange Handbook

1

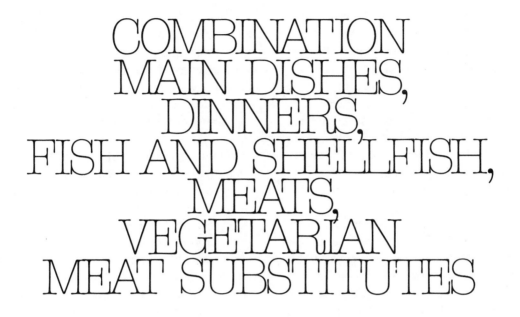

COMBINATION MAIN DISHES, DINNERS, FISH AND SHELLFISH, MEATS, VEGETARIAN MEAT SUBSTITUTES

☐ Canned and frozen main dishes and main dish mixes

☐ Frozen dinners

☐ Canned and frozen fish and shellfish

☐ Canned, frozen, and refrigerated meats

☐ Vegetarian meat substitutes

Prepared main dishes and dinners are convenient and tasty, but trying to calculate exchanges for them is often difficult because you don't know how much of each ingredient is included. Now,

you can stop "guesstimating" exchanges for these items. Instead, consult the listings here for accurate exchanges for popular brands of prepared main dishes, dinners, meats, and fish, calculated from their actual nutrient content.

On evenings when there's just no time to prepare a complete meal from scratch, the extra money you pay for the convenience of prepared foods may be worth it. But first, look at the exchanges for the products you're considering. Is the number of bread and fat exchanges excessive when compared to the number of meat exchanges? Are portions appropriate? Will you be tempted to finish an individually packaged item—even though its exchanges exceed those you're allowed—rather than "waste" the extra amount? Also, consider the presence of extra salt and preservatives. The estimated safe and adequate daily intake of sodium for an adult is 1,100 to 3,300 milligrams (1 to 3.3 grams) per day. Single servings of some prepared main dishes contain 1,000 to 1,500 milligrams of sodium.

The largest section in this chapter, COMBINATION MAIN DISHES, contains main dish items that combine ingredients from different exchange groups. Canned main dishes include chili, hash, stew, and pasta dishes such as spaghetti and meatballs. These items usually contain meat, fat, and bread exchanges; some also contain vegetable exchanges. Be sure to consider all of these when planning the rest of your meal. Since many of these items will contain all your allowed bread and fat exchanges as well as some or all of your meat exchanges, you won't want to add more of these exchanges to your meal. Fresh vegetables or a salad would be better additions.

Frozen main dishes are also combinations of meat, fat, bread, and vegetable exchanges. You'll find beef, chicken, pork, and turkey dishes listed here, as well as Mexican foods, pizza, pot pies, and pasta dishes with meat or cheese—anything that contains a meat exchange item in combination with other foods. (Fish items are listed separately.) Some of these foods also include additional bread exchanges in the form of potatoes or stuffing.

Main dish mixes are listed here as *prepared*—after you add the suggested meat or vegetables. Some of these are simply flavoring packets—you add most of the ingredients yourself. But when average calculated values for the final product could be obtained, we included

them here as a convenience. (Other main-dish seasoning mixes for which prepared values could not be obtained can be found in Chapter 7.)

Frozen dinners, consisting of a main dish and one or more side dishes, may contain all your allowed exchanges for a meal except milk and fruit. Some may exceed your allowed exchanges in one category or another, and you may find you can work them into your meal plan only by omitting side dishes or by eating only part of the main dish.

Canned and frozen fish and shellfish items are listed in a separate section. Canned items include clams, tuna, salmon, sardines, and oysters. You'll find surprising differences in such items as canned salmon (red salmon contains more fat than pink) and canned tuna (varieties packed in oil contain up to two fat exchanges per serving, while those packed in water have no fat exchanges). Frozen fish also varies greatly. Plain fish filets have exchanges similar to those of fresh fish, while items such as shellfish crêpes or fritters, fish cakes, and fried fish filets contain substantial bread and fat exchanges.

In the section labeled MEATS you'll find canned, frozen, and refrigerated brand-name meats such as chicken, turkey, and ham. Although exchanges for these items can be found in other exchange lists, portion sizes for prepackaged items may not always correspond to those listed. For your convenience, we've calculated these items per piece, per can, or per the manufacturer's suggested serving size.

Finally, we've included a section on vegetarian meat substitutes. Like meats, these foods are high in protein and contain both meat and fat exchanges. However, these soy and grain products also contain carbohydrate—enough, in some instances, to count as half a bread exchange.

Product Name	Serving Size	Calories	Exchanges

COMBINATION MAIN DISHES

■ Canned

Beef,

Creamed dried,
Hormel Short Orders . . . . 7½ oz. . . . . 160 . . . . ½ B, 1 M, 1½ F

Goulash,
Heinz . . . . 7½ oz. . . . . 240 . . . 1 B, 1 M, 1 V, 2 F
Hormel Short Orders . . . . 7½ oz. . . . . 230 . . . . 1 B, 2 M, 1 F

Stew,
Armour . . . . 8 oz. . . . . 210 . . . . . 1 B, 1 M, ½ V, 1½ F
Dia-Mel . . . . 8 oz. . . . . 200 . . . 1 B, 1½ M, ½ V, 1 F
Dinty Moore . . . . 7½ oz. . . . . 180 . . . . . . 1 B, 1½ M, ½ F
Dinty Moore Short Orders . . . . . 7½ oz. . . . . 170 . . . . . . 1 B, 1½ M, ½ F
Featherweight . . . . 7½ oz. . . . . 220 . . . . 1½ B, 1½ M, ½ V, ½ F
Heinz . . . . 7¼ oz. . . . . 210 . . . . 1 B, 1 M, 1 V, 1 F
Libby's . . . . 7½ oz. . . . . 160 . . . . 1 B, 1 M, ½ V, ½ F
Swanson . . . . 7½ oz. . . . . 150 . . . . . ½ B, 1 M, ½ V, 1 F

Burritos, beef, *Hormel* . . . . 4 oz. . . . . 220 . . . . 2 B, 1 M, 1 F

Chicken,

with Dumplings,
Featherweight . . . . 7½ oz. . . . . 160 . . . . . . 1½ B, 1 M
Swanson . . . . 7½ oz. . . . . 220 . . . 1½ B, 1 M, 1½ F

à la King, *Swanson* . . . . 5¼ oz. . . . . 180 . . . . . ½ B, 1 M, 2 F

Stew,
Dia-Mel . . . . 8 oz. . . . . 150 . . . . . 1½ B, 1 M
Featherweight . . . . 7½ oz. . . . . 170 . . . . 1 B, 1 M, ½ V, ½ F
Swanson . . . . 7½ oz. . . . . 170 . . . . . 1 B, 1 M, 1 F

with Dumplings, *Heinz* . . . . 7½ oz. . . . . 210 . . . . 1 B, 1 M, 1 V, 1 F

Chili,
Van Camp Chilee Weenee . . . . . . 8 oz. . . . . 290 . . . . . 1½ B, 1½ M, ½ V, 2 F

with Beans,
Armour . . . . 7¾ oz. . . . . 360 . . . . . 1½ B, 1½ M, ½ V, 3½ F
Featherweight . . . . 7½ oz. . . . . 270 . . . . . 1½ B, 1½ M, ½ V, 1½ F
Hormel . . . . 7½ oz. . . . . 320 . . . . . 1½ B, 2 M, 2½ F
Hormel Short Orders . . . . 7½ oz. . . . . 300 . . . . . . 1½ B, 2 M, 2 F
Libby's . . . . 7½ oz. . . . . 270 . . . . . 1½ B, 1 M, ½ V, 2 F
Van Camp . . . . 8 oz. . . . . 340 . . . . . 1½ B, 1½ M, ½ V, 3 F
Hot, *Hormel Short Orders* . . . . . . 7½ oz. . . . . 300 . . . . . . 1½ B, 2 M, 2 F
Texas, *Armour* . . . . 7¾ oz. . . . . 340 . . . . 1½ B, 1 M, ½ V, 3½ F

without Beans,
Armour . . . . 7½ oz. . . . . 390 . . . . . . ½ B, 1½ M, ½ V, 5½ F

Product Name	Serving Size	Calories	Exchanges
Hormel	7½ oz.	340	½ B, 3 M, 3 F
Hormel Short Orders	7½ oz.	370	½ B, 2 M, 5 F
Libby's	7½ oz.	390	½ B, 1½ M, ½ V, 5½ F
Van Camp	8 oz.	390	½ B, 1½ M, ½ V, 5½ F
Texas, Armour	7½ oz.	430	½ B, 1½ M, ½ V, 6½ F
Con carne with beans,			
Campbell's low sodium	7¾ oz.	310	2 B, 2 M, 1½ F
Heinz	7¾ oz.	350	1 B, 1½ M, 2 V, 3 F
Swanson	7¾ oz.	310	2 B, 2 M, 1½ F
Chili and macaroni,			
Hormel Short Orders, Chili Mac	7½ oz.	200	1 B, 1 M, 1½ F
in Sauce, Heinz	7½ oz.	250	1½ B, 1 M, 2 F
Chow mein,			
Beef,			
La Choy	¾ cup	70	½ M, 1 V, ½ F
La Choy Bi-Pack	¾ cup	60	½ M, 1 V
Beef Pepper Oriental,			
La Choy	¾ cup	90	½ B, ½ M, 1 V
La Choy Bi-Pack	¾ cup	70	½ M, 1 V, ½ F
Chicken,			
La Choy	¾ cup	80	½ M, 1 V, ½ F
La Choy Bi-Pack	¾ cup	70	½ M, 1 V, ½ F
Meatless, La Choy	¾ cup	35	1 V
Pork,			
Hormel Short Orders	7½ oz.	140	½ M, 2½ V, 1 F
La Choy Bi-Pack	¾ cup	90	½ M, 1 V, 1 F
Shrimp,			
La Choy	¾ cup	60	½ M, 1 V
La Choy Bi-Pack	¾ cup	70	½ M, 1 V, ½ F
Vegetable, La Choy Bi-Pack	¾ cup	60	1 V, ½ F
Hash,			
Corned beef,			
Armour	7½ oz.	410	1 B, 2 M, 5 F
Libby's	7½ oz.	400	1½ B, 2 M, 4 F
Mary Kitchen	7½ oz.	400	1½ B, 2½ M, 3½ F
Mary Kitchen Short Orders	7½ oz.	370	1 B, 2½ M, 3½ F
Roast Beef,			
Mary Kitchen	7½ oz.	390	1½ B, 2½ M, 3½ F
Mary Kitchen Short Orders	7½ oz.	370	1½ B, 2 M, 3½ F
Hashed potatoes and beef,			
Dinty Moore Short Orders	7½ oz.	250	1½ B, 1 M, 2 F

Product Name	Serving Size	Calories	Exchanges
Lasagna,			
Hormel Short Orders	7½ oz.	260	1½ B, 1 M, 2½ F
Beef, *Hormel*	10 oz.	370	2 B, 3½ M, 1 F
Macaroni,			
and Beef in tomato sauce,			
Franco-American Beefy Mac	7½ oz.	220	2 B, ½ M, 1 F
Franco-American Beefy O's	7½ oz.	220	2 B, ½ M, 1 F
Heinz	7¼ oz.	200	1 B, 1 M, 1 V, 1 F
and Cheese,			
Franco-American	7¼ oz.	170	1½ B, ½ M, 1 F
Heinz	7½ oz.	190	1½ B, 1 M, ½ F
Hormel Short Orders	7½ oz.	170	1½ B, 1 M, ½ F
Elbow, *Franco-American*	7⅜ oz.	170	1½ B, ½ M, 1 F
in Pizza sauce,			
Franco-American PizzO's	7½ oz.	170	2 B, ½ V, ½ F
Mulligan stew,			
Dinty Moore Short Orders	7½ oz.	230	1 B, 1½ M, 1½ F
Noodles,			
and Beef, *Hormel Short Orders*	7½ oz.	230	1 B, 2 M, 1 F
with Beef and sauce, *Heinz*	7½ oz.	170	1 B, 1 M, 1 F
and Chicken,			
Dinty Moore Short Orders	7½ oz.	210	1 B, 1 M, 2 F
Heinz	7¼ oz.	160	1 B, 1 M, 1 V
and Tuna, *Heinz*	7½ oz.	170	1 B, 1 M, 1 V
Pork brains in milk gravy, *Armour*	2¾ oz.	100	1 M, 1 F
Potatoes,			
Au gratin and bacon, *Hormel Short Orders*	7½ oz.	230	1½ B, 1 M, 1½ F
Scalloped, and ham, *Hormel Short Orders*	7½ oz.	250	1 B, 1 M, 2½ F
Ravioli,			
Beef,			
Dia-Mel	8 oz.	260	2½ B, ½ M, 1½ F
Featherweight	8 oz.	260	2 B, ½ M, ½ V, 2 F
Franco-American	7½ oz.	230	2 B, 1 M, ½ V, ½ F
Franco-American Raviolios	7½ oz.	210	2 B, 1 M, ½ V
Cheese, *Franco-American Raviolios*	7½ oz.	260	2 B, ½ M, 1 V, 1½ F
Sloppy Joes,			
Hormel Short Orders	7½ oz.	340	1 B, 2½ M, 3 F
Beef,			
Armour	7½ oz.	330	1½ B, 1 M, 3½ F
Libby's	⅓ cup	110	½ B, ½ M, 1 F

Product Name	Serving Size	Calories	Exchanges
Pork,			
Armour	7½ oz.	350	1½ B, 1½ M, 3½ F
Libby's	⅓ cup	120	½ B, ½ M, 1½ F
Spaghetti,			
and Beef, *Hormel Short Orders*	7½ oz.	240	1½ B, 1 M, 2 F
and Meatballs,			
Dia-Mel	8 oz.	220	1½ B, 1 M, 1½ F
Featherweight	7½ oz.	200	1½ B, ½ M, ½ V, 1F
Franco-American	7⅜ oz.	210	1½ B, 1 M, 1 F, ½ V
Franco-American SpaghettiO's	7½ oz.	210	1½ B, 1 M, 1 F, ½ V
Hormel Short Orders	7 oz.	210	1½ B, 1 M, 1 F
in Meat sauce,			
Franco-American	7½ oz.	220	1 B, 1 M, 1 V, 1½ F
Heinz	7½ oz.	170	1 B, ½ M, 1 V, 1 F
with Sliced franks in tomato sauce,			
Franco-American SpaghettiO's	7⅜ oz.	220	1½ B, 1 M, 1 F, ½ V
in Tomato sauce with cheese,			
Franco-American	7⅜ oz.	180	2 B, 1 V, ½ F
Franco-American SpaghettiO's	7⅜ oz.	170	2 B, 1 V
Heinz	7½ oz.	160	2 B, ½ F
Sukiyaki, *La Choy Bi-Pack*	¾ cup	70	1 M, ½ V
Tamales,			
Beef,			
Armour, 13½ oz. pkg.	6¾ oz.	350	1½ B, ½ M, ½ V, 4½ F
Armour, 15½ oz. pkg.	7¾ oz.	400	2 B, ½ M, ½ V, 5 F
Hormel Short Orders	7½ oz.	270	1 B, 1 M, 3 F
with Chili gravy, *Old El Paso*	2 tamales	232	1½ B, ½ V, 2½ F
Vegetable stew, *Dinty Moore*	7½ oz.	160	1 B, ½ V, 1½ F

■ Frozen

Product Name	Serving Size	Calories	Exchanges
Beef,			
with Barbeque sauce,			
Pepperidge Farm Deli's	1 piece	270	2 B, 1½ M, 1 F
Chop suey with rice, *Stouffer's*	12 oz.	355	2½ B, 1½ M, 1 V, 1½ F
Chow mein,			
Green Giant Twin Pouch	10 oz.	260	2 B, 1 M, ½ V, 1 F
Van de Kamp's Chinese Classics	11 oz.	370	1½ B, 2½ M, 1 V, 2 F
Creamed chipped,			
Stouffer's	5½ oz.	235	½ B, 1 M, 2½ F, ½ Mk
Swanson	10½ oz.	330	1 B, 2½ M, 3 F
Oriental with vegetables and rice,			
Stouffer's Lean Cuisine	8⅝ oz.	280	2 B, 2 M, 1 V

Product Name	Serving Size	Calories	Exchanges
Sliced,			
with Brown sauce in pastry, *Pepperidge Farm Deli's*	1 piece	270	2 B, 1 M, 2 F
with Gravy and whipped potatoes, *Swanson*	8 oz.	200	1 B, 2 M, ½ F
with Whipped potatoes, *Swanson Hungry Man*	12¼ oz.	300	1½ B, 3½ M
and Spinach-stuffed pasta shells with tomato sauce, *Stouffer's*	9 oz.	290	1½ B, 2 M, 1 V, 1 F
Stew,			
Green Giant Boil-in-Bag	9 oz.	180	1½ B, 1 M, ½ V
Stouffer's	10 oz.	310	1 B, 2½ M, ½ V, 2 F
Stroganoff,			
with Noodles, *Green Giant Twin Pouch*	9 oz.	340	2½ B, 2 M, 1 F
with Parsley noodles, *Stouffer's*	9¾ oz.	390	2 B, 2½ M, 2½ F
Teriyaki with rice and vegetables, *Stouffer's*	10 oz.	365	2 B, 2½ M, 1 F, 1 Fr
and Vegetables Szechwan with rice, *Van de Kamp's Chinese Classics*	11 oz.	370	2 B, 2 M, 1 V, 2 F
Burritos,			
Beef,			
El Charrito	1 burrito	810	5½ B, 2 M, 7 F
Fallowfield's Mexican Way	1 burrito	750	5 B, 2 M, 6½ F
and Bean with chili salsa, *Van de Kamp's*	6 oz.	280	3 B, 1 M, ½ F
Red hot, *El Charrito*	1 burrito	340	2½ B, 1 M, 2½ F
Crispy fried, and guacamole, *Van de Kamp's Mexican Classics*	6 oz.	350	3 B, 1 M, 2 F
Green chili beef and bean, *El Charrito*	1 burrito	350	3 B, 1 M, 2 F
Red chili beef and bean,			
El Charrito	1 burrito	350	3 B, 1 M, 2 F
Prefried, *El Charrito*	1 burrito	350	2½ B, 1 M, 2½ F
Red hot,			
El Charrito	1 burrito	350	3 B, 1 M, 2 F
Beef and bean, *El Charrito*	1 burrito	390	2½ B, 1 M, 3½ F
Prefried, *El Charrito*	1 burrito	360	2½ B, 1 M, 3 F
Rolls,			
Beef, *El Charrito*	1 entree	820	8 B, 1½ M, 4½ F
Quesorito, *El Charrito*	1 entree	830	6½ B, 1½ M, 7 F
Ranchorito, *El Charrito*	1 entree	770	6 B, 2 M, 5½ F
Cabbage rolls, stuffed, *Green Giant*	7 oz.	200	1 B, 1 M, ½ V, 1 F
Cannelloni, *Stouffer's Lean Cuisine,*			
Beef and pork with Mornay sauce	9⅞ oz.	240	½ B, 2 M, ½ V, 1 F, ½ Mk

Product Name	Serving Size	Calories	Exchanges
Cheese with tomato sauce	9½ oz.	260	1 B, 2½ M, ½ V, ½ F
Cheese,			
Soufflé, *Stouffer's*	6 oz.	355	1 B, 2 M, 4 F
Stuffed pasta shells with meat sauce, *Stouffer's*	9 oz.	320	1 B, 3 M, ½ V, 1½ F
Chicken,			
Au gratin, *Weaver*	6 oz.	210	1½ B, 1½ M, ½ F
and Broccoli with rice in cheese sauce, *Green Giant Twin Pouch*	10 oz.	370	1½ B, 3 M, 1 V, 1½ F
Cacciatore with spaghetti, *Stouffer's*	11¼ oz.	310	1½ B, 2½ M, 1 V, 1 F
Cantonese, almond, with rice, *Van de Kamp's Chinese Classics*	11 oz.	430	2½ B, 3 M, 2 F
Chow mein,			
Green Giant Twin Pouch	9 oz.	220	2 B, 1 M, 1 V
Van de Kamp's Chinese Classics	11 oz.	380	2 B, 3 M, 1 V, 1 F
with Rice, *Stouffer's* Lean Cuisine	11¼ oz.	240	2 B, 1½ M, 1 V
without Noodles, *Stouffer's.*	8 oz.	145	½ B, 1½ M, 1 V
Creamed, *Stouffer's*	6½ oz.	300	2 M, 3½ F, ½ Mk
Croquettes, *Weaver*	2 oz.	160	½ B, 1 M, 1½ F
(Gravy)	0.9 oz.	15	free in moderation
Divan, *Stouffer's*	8½ oz.	335	2 M, 1 V, 3 F, ½ Mk
Fried,			
Assorted pieces, *Swanson*	3¼ oz.*	290	1 B, 2 M, 2½ F
Breast portions, *Swanson*	3¼ oz.*	250	1 B, 2 M, 1½ F
Breasts, *Weaver* Batter Dipped	3.7 oz.*	280	½ B, 2½ M, 2½ F
Breasts, *Weaver Dutch Frye*	3.7 oz.*	280	1 B, 2½ M, 1½ F
Dark portions, *Swanson Hungry Man*	10¾ oz.*	590	2½ B, 3½ M, 5 F
Drumsticks, *Weaver* Dutch Frye	3.4 oz.*	240	1 B, 2 M, 1½ F
Italian style, *Weaver*	3.5 oz.*	250	1 B, 2 M, 1½ F
Mini-drums, crispy, *Weaver*	1 piece (0.6 oz.)	45	½ M, ½ F
Mini-drums, *Herbs 'N Spice, Weaver*	1 piece (0.6 oz.)	45	½ M, ½ F
Party pack, *Weaver* Batter Dipped	1.5 oz.*	130	½ B, ½ M, 1½ F
Party pack, *Weaver* Dutch Frye	1.5 oz.*	130	½ B, ½ M, 1½ F
Rounds, with cheese, *Weaver Rondelets*	3.0 oz.	210	1 B, 1½ M, 1½ F
Rounds, Italian, *Weaver Rondelets*	3.0 oz.	230	½ B, 1 M, 2 F

*Edible portion.

Product Name	Serving Size	Calories	Exchanges
Rounds, original flavor, *Weaver Rondelets*	3.0 oz.	210	1 B, 1½ M, 1½ F
Sticks, *Weaver*	1.0 oz.	70	½ M, 1 F
Take-out style, *Swanson*	3¼ oz.*	270	1 B, 2 M, 2 F
Thighs and drumsticks, *Swanson*	3¼ oz.*	280	1 B, 2½ M, 1½ F
Thighs/Drums, *Weaver Batter Dipped*	3.5 oz.*	260	½ B, 2 M, 2½ F
Thighs/Drums, *Weaver Dutch Frye*	3.5 oz.*	260	½ B, 2 M, 2½ F
with Whipped potatoes, *Swanson*	7¼ oz.*	400	2 B, 2 M, 3½ F
White portions, *Swanson Hungry Man*	11¾ oz.*	720	3½ B, 5½ M, 4 F
Wing sections, nibbles, *Swanson*	3¼ oz.*	300	1 B, 2 M, 3 F
Glazed, with vegetable rice, *Stouffer's Lean Cuisine*	8½ oz.	270	3 M, 1½ B
à la King, *Weight Watchers*	9 oz.	230	½ B, 2½ M, ½ V, ½ Mk
with Rice, *Stouffer's*	9½ oz.	330	2 B, 1½ M, ½ V, 1½ F, ½ Mk
and Noodles, *Green Giant Twin Pouch*	9 oz.	370	2½ B, 1½ M, 2½ F
Escalloped, *Stouffer's*	5¾ oz.	250	1 B, 1½ M, 2 F
Paprikash with egg noodles, *Stouffer's*	10½ oz.	385	2 B, 3½ M, 1 F
Patties, Breaded, and fries, *Mrs. Paul's*	8½ oz.	390	3½ B, 2 M, 1 F
Light batter, and fries, *Mrs. Paul's*	8½ oz.	420	3 B, 1½ M, 3 F
and Pea pods, *Green Giant Twin Pouch*	10 oz.	330	2 B, 1½ M, 1 V, 1½ F
Salad, savory, in pastry, *Pepperidge Farm Deli's*	1 piece	340	1½ B, 1½ M, 3½ F
Sticks, breaded, and fries, *Mrs. Paul's*	8½ oz.	420	3½ B, 2 M, 1½ F
Stuffed pasta shells with cheese sauce, *Stouffer's*	9 oz.	400	1½ B, 3 M, 3 F
Turnovers, *Weaver*	4.0 oz.	340	2 B, 1 M, 3½ F
in White wine sauce, *Swanson*	8¼ oz.	350	½ B, 3 M, 3½ F
and Vegetables with vermicelli, *Stouffer's Lean Cuisine*	12¾ oz.	270	2 B, 2 M, 1 V
Chili con carne with beans, *Stouffer's*	8¾ oz.	270	1½ B, 2 M, ½ V, 1 F

*Edible portion.

Product Name	Serving Size	Calories	Exchanges
Weight Watchers	10 oz.	290	1½ B, 3 M, 1 V
Crêpes,			
Chicken with mushroom sauce, *Stouffer's*	8¼ oz.	390	1 B, 3 M, 2½ F, ½ Mk
Ham and asparagus, *Stouffer's*	6¼ oz.	325	1 B, 2 M, 1 V, 2½ F
Ham and swiss cheese, *Stouffer's*	7½ oz.	410	1½ B, 3 M, 3 F
Spinach, *Stouffer's*	9½ oz.	415	1½ B, 2 M, 1 V, 4 F
Egg rolls Cantonese, *Van de Kamp's Chinese Classics*	10½ oz.	550	4 B, 2 M, 1 V, 3 F
Eggs, scrambled,			
with Bacon and cheese in pastry, *Pepperidge Farm Deli's*	4 oz.	290	1½ B, 1 M, 3 F
and Sausage with hash brown potatoes, *Swanson*	6¼ oz.	430	1 B, 1½ M, 6 F
Enchilada,			
Beef,			
Van de Kamp's, 7½ oz. pkg.	7½ oz.	250	1½ B, 1 M, 2 F
Van de Kamp's, 8½ oz. pkg.	8½ oz.	340	2 B, 2 M, 2 F
Shredded, *El Charrito*	1 entree	640	5 B, 2 M, 4 F
Shredded, *Van de Kamp's Mexican Classics*	5½ oz.	180	1 B, 1½ M, ½ F
Cheese,			
El Charrito	1 entree	630	5 B, 2 M, 4 F
Van de Kamp's, 7½ oz. pkg.	7½ oz.	270	1½ B, 1 M, 2½ F
Van de Kamp's, 8½ oz. pkg.	8½ oz.	370	2 B, 1½ M, 3½ F
Ranchero, *Van de Kamp's Mexican Classics*	5½ oz.	252	1½ B, 1 M, 2 F
Chicken,			
El Charrito	1 entree	520	4 B, 2 M, 3 F
Van de Kamp's	7½ oz.	250	1½ B, 1 M, 2 F
with Sour cream sauce, *Van de Kamp's Mexican Classics*	5½ oz.	420	2 B, 1 M, 5 F
Green pepper, stuffed,			
Green Giant	7 oz.	220	1 B, 1 M, ½ V, 2 F
with Beef in tomato sauce, *Stouffer's*	7¾ oz.	225	1 B, 1 M, 1 V, 1½ F
Hash, roast beef, *Stouffer's*	5¾ oz.	265	2 M, 1 B, 2 F
Lasagna,			
Green Giant Boil-in-Bag	9 oz.	310	2½ B, 1 M, 1 V, 1 F
Stouffer's Single Serving	10½ oz.	385	2 B, 3 M, 1 V, 1 F
Beef and mushroom, *Van de Kamp's Italian Classics*	11 oz.	430	1 B, 2½ M, ½ V, 3 F
Chicken, *Green Giant*	12 oz.	640	2 B, 3½ M, 1 V, 4 F, 1 Mk

Product Name	Serving Size	Calories	Exchanges
and Garlic roll, *Swanson Hungry Man*	12¾ oz.	540	3 B, 2 M, ½ V, 4½ F
Italian sausage, *Van de Kamp's Italian Classics*	11 oz.	440	2 B, 3 M, ½ V, 2½ F
with Meat, *Swanson Hungry Man*	12¾ oz.	480	4 B, 2 M, ½ V, 2 F
with Meat sauce, *Green Giant*	12 oz.	470	2½ B, 2 M, 1 V, 3½ F
Spinach,			
Green Giant	12 oz.	370	2½ B, 2 M, ½ V, 1½ F
Van de Kamp's Italian Classics	11 oz.	400	2 B, 2½ M, 1 V, 2 F
in Tomato sauce, *Swanson*	13¼ oz.	480	3 B, 2 M, 1 V, 3 F
with Veal, tomato sauce, and cheese, *Weight Watchers*	12¾ oz.	380	2 B, 2½ M, 2 V, 1 F
Zucchini, *Stouffer's Lean Cuisine*	11 oz.	240	1½ B, 2½ M, ½ V
Linguini with clam sauce, *Stouffer's*	10½ oz.	285	2½ B, 1½ M, 1 F
Macaroni and beef with tomatoes, *Stouffer's*	5¾ oz.	190	1 B, 1 M, 1 F, 1 V
Macaroni and cheese,			
Green Giant Boil-in-Bag	9 oz.	290	2½ B, 1 M, 1½ F
Stouffer's	6 oz.	260	1 B, 1 M, 2 F, ½ Mk
Swanson	12 oz.	440	3 B, 1½ M, 3½ F
Van de Kamp's	5 oz.	150	1½ B, ½ M, ½ F
Meatballs with brown gravy and whipped potatoes, *Swanson*	9¼ oz.	320	1½ B, 1½ M, 3 F
Meatball stew, *Stouffer's Lean Cuisine*	10 oz.	240	1 B, 2½ M, 1 V
Meatloaf with tomato sauce and whipped potatoes, *Swanson*	9 oz.	340	2 B, 1½ M, 3 F
Mexican-style pastry, *Pepperidge Farm Deli's*	1 piece	270	2 B, 1 M, 2 F
Omelets,			
with Cheese sauce and ham, *Swanson*	7 oz.	370	1 B, 2½ M, 3½ F
Spanish style, *Swanson*	7¾ oz.	240	1 B, 1 M, 2½ F
Western style in pastry, *Pepperidge Farm Deli's*	1 piece	290	2 B, ½ M, 3 F
Pizza,			
Canadian-style bacon,			
Celeste, 8 oz. pkg.	1 pizza	490	3½ B, 2½ M, 2½ F
Celeste, 19 oz. pkg.	¼ pizza	290	2 B, 2 M, 1 F
Cheese,			
Celeste, 7 oz. pkg.	1 pizza	470	4 B, 2½ M, 1½ F
Celeste, 19 oz. pkg.	¼ pizza	310	2 B, 1½ M, 2 F
Weight Watchers	6 oz.	370	2 B, 3 M, 1½ F
French bread, *Stouffer's*	5⅛ oz.	330	2½ B, 1 M, ½ V, 2 F

Product Name	Serving Size	Calories	Exchanges
Combination,			
Van de Kamp's	5⅞ oz.	310	1½ B, 2 M, 2 F
Chicago style, *Celeste,* 24 oz. pkg.	¼ pizza	370	2½ B, 2 M, 2 F
Deluxe,			
Celeste, 9 oz. pkg.	1 pizza	570	4 B, 2½ M, 3½ F
Celeste, 23.5 oz. pkg.	¼ pizza	370	2½ B, 2 M, 2 F
Combination with veal sausage, *Weight Watchers*	7¼ oz.	330	2 B, 3½ M
French bread, *Stouffer's*	6³⁄₁₆ oz.	400	2½ B, 1½ M, 1 V, 2½ F
Sicilian style, *Celeste,* 26 oz. pkg.	¼ pizza	420	3 B, 1½ M, 3 F
Hamburger, French bread, *Stouffer's*	6⅛ oz.	400	2½ B, 1½ M, ½ V, 3 F
Mexican style, *Van de Kamp's Mexican Classics*	5½ oz.	420	2 B, 1½ M, 4½ F
Mushroom, French bread, *Stouffer's*	6 oz.	340	2½ B, 1 M, 1 V, 2 F
Pepperoni,			
Celeste, 7¼ oz. pkg.	1 pizza	570	4 B, 2½ M, 3½ F
Celeste, 20 oz. pkg.	¼ pizza	350	2½ B, 1 M, 2½ F
Van de Kamp's	5½ oz.	370	2½ B, 2 M, 2 F
Chicago style, *Celeste,* 24 oz. pkg.	¼ pizza	380	2½ B, 1½ M, 3 F
French bread, *Stouffer's*	5⅝ oz.	410	2½ B, 1 M, ½ V, 3½ F
Sausage,			
Celeste, 8 oz. pkg.	1 pizza	530	4 B, 2 M, 3½ F
Celeste, 22 oz. pkg.	¼ pizza	360	2½ B, 1½ M, 2½ F
Chicago style, *Celeste,* 24 oz. pkg.	¼ pizza	390	2½ B, 2 M, 2½ F
French bread, *Stouffer's*	6 oz.	420	2½ B, 1½ M, ½ V, 3½ F
and Mushroom, *Celeste,* 9 oz. pkg.	1 pizza	560	4 B, 2½ M, 3½ F
and Mushroom, *Celeste,* 24 oz. pkg.	¼ pizza	370	2½ B, 2 M, 2 F
and Mushroom, French bread, *Stouffer's*	6¼ oz.	395	2½ B, 1½ M, 1 V, 2½ F
Suprema,			
Celeste, 10 oz. pkg.	1 pizza	590	3½ B, 3½ M, 3½ F
Celeste, 24 oz. pkg.	¼ pizza	360	2½ B, 1½ M, 2½ F
without Meat, *Celeste,* 8 oz. pkg.	1 pizza	440	3½ B, 2 M, 2 F
without Meat, *Celeste,* 20 oz. pkg.	¼ pizza	280	2 B, 1 M, 1 F
Veal sausage, *Weight Watchers*	6¾ oz.	350	2 B, 2½ M, 1 V, 1 F
Vegetable supreme, *Weight Watchers*	7¼ oz.	400	2 B, 3 M, 1 V, 1½ F

Product Name	Serving Size	Calories	Exchanges
Pizza-style pastry,			
Pepperidge Farm Deli's	1 piece	290	2 B, ½ M, 3 F
Pot pie,			
Beef,			
Stouffer's	10 oz.	550	2 B, 2 M, 1 V, 6 F
Swanson	8 oz.	400	2½ B, 1 M, 4 F
Swanson Hungry Man	16 oz.	720	4 B, 3 M, 1 V, 5½ F
Chicken,			
Stouffer's	10 oz.	500	2½ B, 2 M, 1 V, 4 F
Swanson	8 oz.	440	3 B, 1 M, 4 F
Swanson Hungry Man	16 oz.	730	4 B, 3 M, 1 V, 6 F
Van de Kamp's	7½ oz.	520	3 B, 1½ M, 5 F
Macaroni and cheese, *Swanson*	7 oz.	210	1½ B, 1 M, 1 F
Steak burger,			
Swanson Hungry Man	16 oz.	730	3½ B, 3 M, 1 V, 7 F
Turkey,			
Stouffer's	10 oz.	460	2 B, 2 M, 1 V, 4 F
Swanson	8 oz.	430	2½ B, 1 M, 4½ F
Swanson Hungry Man	16 oz.	730	4 B, 3 M, 1 V, 6 F
Reuben in pastry,			
Pepperidge Farm Deli's	1 piece	360	1½ B, 1½ M, 4 F
Salisbury steak,			
Green Giant Boil-in-Bag	9 oz.	410	1 B, 4 M, 2½ F
with Crinkle-cut potatoes,			
Swanson	5½ oz.	350	2 B, 1½ M, 3 F
Swanson Hungry Man	12½ oz.	640	2½ B, 4 M, 5½ F
in Gravy,			
Green Giant	7 oz.	220	1 B, 2 M, 1 F
Swanson	10 oz.	410	1 B, 3½ M, 3½ F
with Italian-style vegetables and sauce, *Stouffer's Lean Cuisine*	9⅝ oz.	270	3 M, 2 V, 1 F
with Onion gravy, *Stouffer's*	6 oz.	250	½ B, 3 M, 1 F
Short ribs of beef with vegetable gravy, *Stouffer's*	5¾ oz.	350	4 M, ½ V, 2½ F
Spaghetti,			
with Beef and mushroom sauce, *Stouffer's Lean Cuisine*	11½ oz.	280	2 B, 1½ M, 2 V
with Breaded veal, *Swanson*	9 oz.	310	2 B, 1½ M, 2 F
and Meatballs, *Green Giant Twin Pouch*	10 oz.	400	3½ B, 1 M, ½ V, 2 F
with Meat sauce, *Stouffer's*	14 oz.	445	3 B, 2 M, 2 V, 1½ F
Steak and green peppers,			
Green Giant Twin Pouch	9 oz.	280	2 B, 2½ M, ½ V
in Oriental style sauce, *Swanson*	8½ oz.	180	½ B, 2½ M, ½ V

Product Name	Serving Size	Calories	Exchanges
with Rice, *Stouffer's*	12 oz.	355	2 B, 2½ M, 1 V, 1 F
Swedish meatballs with parsley noodles, *Stouffer's*	11 oz.	475	3 M, 2 B, 4 F
Taquitos, shredded beef with guacamole, *Van de Kamp's Mexican Classics*	8 oz.	490	3 B, 1½ M, 4½ F
Tostada, beef supreme, *Van de Kamp's Mexican Classics*	8½ oz.	530	2½ B, 3 M, 4½ F
Tuna noodle casserole, *Stouffer's*	5¾ oz.	200	1 B, 1 M, ½ V, 1 F
Turkey,			
Breast filets with cheese, *Land O' Lakes*	5 oz.	300	1 B, 3½ M, 1 F
Casserole with gravy and dressing,			
Stouffer's	9¾ oz.	370	2 B, 2½ M, ½ V, 2 F
Swanson	9¼ oz.	310	1½ B, 3½ M
and Whipped potatoes, *Swanson*	8¾ oz.	220	1½ B, 2 M
and Whipped potatoes, *Swanson Hungry Man*	13¼ oz.	370	2½ B, 3½ M
Ham, and cheese in pastry, *Pepperidge Farm Deli's*	1 piece	270	1½ B, 1½ M, 2 F
Slices in gravy with white and wild rice, *Green Giant Twin Pouch*	9 oz.	410	2½ B, 2½ M, 2 F
Tetrazzini, *Stouffer's*	6 oz.	240	1 B, 1½ M, 2 F
Welsh rarebit, *Stouffer's*	5 oz.	355	½ B, 1 M, 5 F, ½ Mk
Ziti macaroni with veal, tomato sauce, and cheese, *Weight Watchers*	12½ oz.	340	2½ B, 2 M, 1 V, ½ F

■ **Mixes**

Product Name	Serving Size	Calories	Exchanges
Beef noodle, *Hamburger Helper*	⅕ pkg. prepared	320	1½ B, 2½ M, 1½ F
Beef romanoff, *Hamburger Helper*	⅕ pkg. prepared	340	2 B, 2 M, 2 F
Beef stew, *Durkee*	1 cup prepared	379	1 B, 2½ M, ½ V, 3½ F
Cheeseburger macaroni, *Hamburger Helper*	⅕ pkg. prepared	360	2 B, 2½ M, 2 F
Chili,			
Texas style, *Durkee*	½ cup prepared	386	1 B, 3 M, ½ V, 3 F
Tomato, *Hamburger Helper*	⅕ pkg. prepared	320	2 B, 2 M, 1½ F
Chop suey, *Durkee*	¾ cup prepared	222	½ B, 2½ M, ½ V, 1 F
Ground beef, seasoned,			
Durkee	½ cup prepared	327	½ B, 3 M, 3 F
with Onion, *Durkee*	½ cup prepared	329	½ B, 3 M, 3 F
Hamburger,			
Hash, *Hamburger Helper*	⅕ pkg. prepared	300	1½ B, 2 M, 2 F
Seasoning, *Durkee*	½ cup prepared	332	3½ M, 3 F
Stew, *Hamburger Helper*	⅕ pkg. prepared	290	1½ B, 2 M, 1½ F
Lasagna, *Hamburger Helper*	⅕ pkg. prepared	330	2 B, 2 M, ½ V, 1½ F

Product Name	Serving Size	Calories	Exchanges
Macaroni and cheese,			
Creamettes	2 oz.	220	3 B, ½ M
Golden Grain	¾ cup prepared	200	2½ B, ½ M
Lipton	½ cup prepared	210	1½ B, ½ M, 2 F
Meatball, seasoned, Italian, *Durkee*	½ cup prepared	309	3 M, 3 F
Pizza dish, *Hamburger Helper*	⅕ pkg. prepared	340	2 B, 2 M, ½ V, 1½ F
Potatoes au gratin, *Hamburger Helper*	⅕ pkg. prepared	320	2 B, 2 M, 1½ F
Quiche, *Pour-A-Quiche,*			
Bacon and onion	4½ oz.	230	½ B, 1½ M, 2½ F
Spinach and onion	4⅓ oz.	220	1½ M, ½ V, 2½ F
Three-cheese	4⅓ oz.	230	2 M, 2½ F
Rice oriental, *Hamburger Helper*	⅕ pkg. prepared	340	2 B, 2 M, ½ V, 1½ F
Sloppy Joe,			
Durkee	½ cup prepared	290	½ B, 2½ M, ½ V, 2½ F
Pizza flavor, *Durkee*	½ cup prepared	298	½ B, 2½ M, ½ V, 2½ F
Spaghetti, *Hamburger Helper*	⅕ pkg. prepared	330	2 B, 2 M, ½ V, 1½ F
Taco seasoning, *Durkee*	½ cup prepared	320	3 M, 3½ F
Tamale pie, *Hamburger Helper*	⅕ pkg. prepared	370	2½ B, 2 M, ½ V, 1½ F
Tuna casserole, *Tuna Helper,*			
with Country Dumplings and Noodles	⅕ pkg. prepared	230	2 B, 1½ M, ½ F
with Creamy Noodles	⅕ pkg. prepared	280	2 B, 1½ M, 1½ F
with Noodles and Cheese Sauce	⅕ pkg. prepared	230	2 B, 1½ M, ½ F

DINNERS (FROZEN)

Product Name	Serving Size	Calories	Exchanges
Beef,			
Burgundy, *Armour Dinner Classics*	10½ oz.	330	1 B, 3½ M, 1 V, ½ F
Sirloin, in mushroom sauce, with green beans and cauliflower, *Weight Watchers*	13 oz.	410	½ B, 4 M, 2 V, 2 F
Steak, in green pepper and mushroom sauce, with carrots, *Weight Watchers*	9¾ oz.	340	3 M, 2 V, 3 F
Chicken,			
Fricassee, *Armour Dinner Classics*	11¾ oz,	330	1½ B, 3 M, 1 V, ½ F
Oriental, in ginger sauce, with oriental vegetables and rice, *Weight Watchers*	9½ oz.	240	1½ B, 2 M, 1 V
Parmigiana, with Italian green beans, *Weight Watchers*	7¾ oz.	220	3 M, 1½ V
Patty, southern fried, with vegetable medley, *Weight Watchers*	6¾ oz.	260	½ B, 3 M, ½ V, 1 F
Sliced, in celery sauce, with peas and onions, *Weight Watchers*	8½ oz.	230	½ B, 3 M, 1 V

Product Name	Serving Size	Calories	Exchanges
Cod Almondine, *Armour*			
Dinner Classics	12 oz.	380	2½ B, 2½ M, ½ V, 1 F
Enchilada,			
El Charrito	1 dinner	580	4 B, 1½ M, 5 F
Beef, *Van de Kamp's*	12 oz.	390	3 B, 1½ M, 2½ F
Cheese,			
El Charrito	1 dinner	540	4 B, 1½ M, 4 F
Van de Kamp's	12 oz.	450	3 B, 2 M, 3 F
Fish			
Batter dipped, *Van de Kamp's*	11 oz.	540	2½ B, 2 M, 5½ F
Filet,			
Van de Kamp's	12 oz.	300	2 B, 3 M
Au gratin with broccoli, *Weight Watchers*	9¼ oz.	200	½ B, 3 M, ½ V
Italian style, in tomato sauce with cheese, and vegetable medley, *Weight Watchers*	9 oz.	180	3 M, 1 V
in Newburg sauce, with peas and onions, *Weight Watchers*	9¼ oz.	190	½ B, 2½ M, 1 V
Oven fried, in seasoned bread crumbs, with vegetable medley, *Weight Watchers*	6¾ oz.	220	½ B, 3 M, ½ V, ½ F
Flounder with lemon-flavored bread crumbs and vegetable medley, *Weight Watchers*	6½	140	½ B, 2 M, ½ V
Haddock with stuffing and Italian green beans, *Weight Watchers*	7 oz.	210	½ B, 3 M, ½ V
Lasagna, *Armour Dinner Classics*	10 oz.	370	2½ B, 1 M, 1 V, 2½ F
Mexican style,			
El Charrito	1 dinner	650	5 B, 1½ M, 5 F
Van de Kamp's	11½ oz.	421	3 B, 2 M, 2½ F
Combination	11 oz.	430	3 B, 2½ M, 2 F
Ocean perch with lemon-flavored bread crumbs and broccoli, *Weight Watchers*	6½ oz.	160	½ B, 2 M, ½ V
Queso, *El Charrito*	1 dinner	470	5 B, ½ M, 2½ F
Salisbury steak, *Armour*			
Dinner Classics	11 oz.	480	2½ B, 2 M, ½ V, 4 F
Saltillo, *El Charrito*	1 dinner	530	5 B, ½ M, 3½ F
Seafood newburg, *Armour*			
Dinner Classics	10 oz.	260	1½ B, 1 M, 1 V, 1½ F
Shrimp, *Van de Kamp's*	10 oz.	370	2½ B, 1½ M, 2½ F
Sirloin tip, *Armour Dinner Classics*	11 oz.	380	1½ B, 3½ M, 1 V, 1 F
Sole in lemon sauce, with peas and onions, *Weight Watchers*	9¼ oz.	200	½ B, 2½ M, 1½ V
Stuffed green peppers, *Armour Dinner Classics*	12 oz.	420	2½ B, 1 M, ½ V, 4 F

Product Name	Serving Size	Calories	Exchanges
Swedish meatballs, *Armour*			
Dinner Classics	11½ oz.	540	2½ B, 2½ M, ½ V, 5 F
Teriyaki steak, *Armour*			
Dinner Classics	10 oz.	360	1½ B, 3 M, 1 V, 1½ F
Turkey,			
Sliced, with gravy and stuffing, and carrots and broccoli, *Weight Watchers*	15¼ oz.	390	1½ B, 4 M, 2 V
Tetrazzini, with cheese, mushrooms, and red peppers, *Weight Watchers*	10 oz.	310	1½ B, 3 M, ½ V, ½ F
Veal,			
Parmigiana,			
Armour Dinner Classics	10¾ oz.	370	2 B, 1½ M, 1 V, 3 F
with Zucchini in tomato sauce, *Weight Watchers*	9 oz.	250	3 M, 2 V, ½ F
Stuffed pepper in tomato sauce, *Weight Watchers*	11¾ oz.	240	½ B, 3 M, 2 V

FISH AND SHELLFISH

■ Canned

Product Name	Serving Size	Calories	Exchanges
Clams, minced, *Snow's*	6½ oz.	100	2 M
Gefilte fish, *Rokeach*	1 piece	60	1 M
in Natural broth	1 piece	50	1 M
Old Vienna	1 piece	70	½ B, ½ M
Whitefish-pike	1 piece	60	1 M
Salmon,			
Keta, *Bumble Bee*	½ cup	153	3 M
Pink,			
Bumble Bee	½ cup	155	3 M
Del Monte	½ cup	160	3 M
Featherweight	3⅞ oz.	155	3 M
Libby's	3⅞ oz.	155	3 M
Red sockeye,			
Bumble Bee	½ cup	188	3½ M
Del Monte	½ cup	180	3 M
Libby's	3⅞ oz.	190	3½ M
Sardines,			
in Mustard sauce, *Underwood*	1 can (3¾ oz.)	230	2½ M, 2 F
in Soya bean oil, *Underwood*	1 can (3¾ oz.)	380	2½ M, 5½ F
in Tomato sauce,			
Del Monte	½ cup	360	2½ B, 2 M, ½ V, 1½ F
Underwood	1 can (3¾ oz.)	230	2½ M, 2 F

Product Name	Serving Size	Calories	Exchanges

Tuna,

Chunk light in oil,

Bumble Bee	½ can (3.25 oz.)	265	3 M, 2 F
Chicken of the Sea	½ can (3.25 oz.)	225	3 M, 1½ F
Starkist	½ can (3.25 oz.)	225	3 M, 1½ F

Chunk light in water,

Bumble Bee	½ can (3.25 oz.)	117	2 M
Chicken of the Sea	½ can (3.25 oz.)	100	2 M
Featherweight	½ can (3.25 oz.)	105	2 M
Starkist	½ can (3.25 oz.)	100	2 M

Chunk white in oil,
Chicken of the Sea ... ½ can (3.25 oz.) ... 250 ... 3 M, 2 F

Chunk white in water,
low sodium, *Chicken of the Sea* .. ½ can (3.25 oz.) ... 110 ... 2 M

Solid light in oil,
Chicken of the Sea ... ½ can (3.5 oz.) ... 230 ... 3 M, 1½ F

Solid white in oil,

Bumble Bee	½ can (3.5 oz.)	285	3½ M, 2 F
Chicken of the Sea	½ can (3.5 oz.)	225	3 M, 1½ F

Solid white in water,

Bumble Bee	½ can (3.5 oz.)	126	2 M
Chicken of the Sea	½ can (3.5 oz.)	120	2 M
Starkist	½ can (3.5 oz.)	120	2 M

Oysters, whole, *Bumble Bee* ... ½ cup ... 109 ... ½ B, 1½ M

■ Frozen

Clams,

Fried,

Mrs. Paul's	2½ oz.	270	1½ B, 1 M, 2½ F
Sandwich, *Mrs. Paul's*	4½ oz.	420	3½ B, 1 M, 3 F

Fritters, *Mrs. Paul's* ... 3.8 oz. ... 260 ... 2 B, 1 M, 1½ F

Cod, *Today's Catch* ... 4 oz. ... 80 ... 1½ M

Crab,

Crêpes, *Mrs. Paul's*	5½ oz.	240	1½ B, 1 M, 2 F
Deviled, *Mrs. Paul's*	3 oz.	170	1 B, 1 M, 1 F
Miniatures	3½ oz.	220	1 B, 2 M, 1 F

Fritters, *Mrs. Paul's* ... 3.8 oz. ... 250 ... 2 B, ½ M, 2 F

Fish,

Au gratin, *Mrs. Paul's*	5 oz.	250	1½ B, 1 M, 2 F
Cakes, *Mrs. Paul's*	4 oz.	210	1½ B, 1 M, 1 F
Beach Haven	4 oz.	210	1½ B, 1 M, 1 F
Thins	5 oz.	320	2 B, 1 M, 3 F

Product Name	Serving Size	Calories	Exchanges

and Chips,

Mrs. Paul's Light Batter	7 oz.	370	3 B, 1 M, 2½ F
Mrs. Paul's Supreme Light Batter	8½ oz.	450	3 B, 1½ M, 3½ F
Swanson	5 oz.	300	2 B, 1 M, 2½ F
Van de Kamp's Batter Dipped	8 oz.	500	3 B, 1½ M, 5 F

Filets,

Today's Catch	4 oz.	90	1½ M
Van de Kamp's Batter Dipped	6 oz.	440	1½ B, 2 M, 5 F
(Tartar sauce)	1 oz. pkg.	160	3½ F
Divan, Stouffer's Lean Cuisine	12⅜ oz.	270	1 B, 3 M, 1 V
Florentine, Stouffer's Lean Cuisine	9 oz.	230	3 M, 1 V, ½ Mk
Fried, Mrs. Paul's	4 oz.	220	1½ B, 1½ M, 1 F
Fried, Mrs. Paul's Crunchy Light Batter	4½ oz.	350	2½ B, 1 M, 3 F
Fried, Mrs. Paul's Light Batter	3 oz.	150	1 B, 1½ M
Fried, Mrs. Paul's Supreme Light Batter	1 filet	220	1½ B, 1 M, 1½ F
Fried, Van de Kamp's	4 oz.	310	1½ B, 1 M, 3½ F
Portions, fried, Van de Kamp's Batter Dipped	3 oz.	190	1 B, ½ M, 2 F
Sandwich, Mrs. Paul's	4⅛ oz.	200	1½ B, 1½ M, ½ F

Kabobs,

Mrs. Paul's Supreme Light Batter	3.3 oz.	200	1 B, 1 M, 1½ F
Van de Kamp's Batter Dipped	4 oz.	260	1 B, 1 M, 3 F
Van de Kamp's Country Seasoned	4 oz.	290	1 B, 1½ M, 3 F
Parmesan, Mrs. Paul's	5 oz.	220	1½ B, 1 M, 1½ F

Sticks,

Mrs. Paul's	3 oz.	150	1 B, 1 M, ½ F
Mrs. Paul's Crunchy Light Batter	3½ oz.	280	1½ B, 1 M, 2½ F
Van de Kamp's Light and Crispy	3¾ oz.	290	1½ B, 1 M, 3 F

Flounder,

Today's Catch	4 oz.	80	1½ M
Filets, fried, Mrs. Paul's	4 oz.	220	1½ B, 1½ M, 1 F
with Lemon butter, Mrs. Paul's	4¼ oz.	150	½ B, 1½ M, 1 F

Haddock,

Van de Kamp's Batter Dipped	4 oz.	330	1 B, 1½ M, 4 F
Filets, fried, Mrs. Paul's	4 oz.	230	1½ B, 1½ M, 1 F

Product Name	Serving Size	Calories	Exchanges
Halibut, *Van de Kamp's*			
Batter Dipped	4 oz.	270	1 B, 1½ M, 2½ F
Ocean perch filets, fried, *Mrs. Paul's*	3½ oz.	255	1 B, 2 M, 1½ F
Perch,			
Today's Catch	4 oz.	110	2 M
Van de Kamp's Batter Dipped	4 oz.	290	1½ B, 1½ M, 2½ F
Scallops,			
with Batter and cheese,			
Mrs. Paul's	7 oz.	260	½ B, 4 M
Fried, *Mrs. Paul's*	3½ oz.	210	1½ B, 1 M, 1 F
Light Batter	3½ oz.	200	1½ B, 1 M, 1 F
Oriental, with vegetables and			
rice, *Stouffer's Lean Cuisine*	11 oz.	230	1½ B, 2 M, ½ V
and Shrimp mariner with			
rice, *Stouffer's*	10¼ oz.	400	2 B, 2½ M, 2 F, ½ Mk
Seafood platter, combination,			
Mrs. Paul's	9 oz.	510	4 B, 2 M, 3 F
Shrimp,			
Crêpes, *Mrs. Paul's*	5½ oz.	250	1½ B, 1 M, 2 F
Fried, *Mrs. Paul's*	3 oz.	170	1 B, 1 M, 1 F
Fritters, *Mrs. Paul's*	3.8 oz.	240	1½ B, 1 M, 2 F
Sole,			
Today's Catch	4 oz.	80	1½ M
Van de Kamp's Batter Dipped	4 oz.	280	1½ B, 1½ M, 2 F
with Lemon butter, *Mrs. Paul's*	4¼ oz.	160	½ B, 1½ M, 1 F
Tuna fritters, *Mrs. Paul's*	3.8 oz.	270	2 B, 1 M, 2 F

MEATS

■ Canned

Product Name	Serving Size	Calories	Exchanges
Beef steaks, breaded, *Hormel*	4 oz.	370	1½ M, 5 F
Chicken,			
Swanson,			
Chunk	2½ oz.	110	2 M
Chunk style mixing	2½ oz.	130	2 M, ½ F
Chunk white	2½ oz.	110	2 M
Tender Chunk	3 oz.	110	2 M
Corned beef,			
Dinty Moore	3 oz.	190	3½ M
Libby's	2.3 oz.	160	2½ M, ½ F
Ham,			
Oscar Mayer Jubilee	3 oz.	90	1½ M

Product Name	Serving Size	Calories	Exchanges
Tender Chunk	3 oz.	140	2 M, 1 F
Patties, *Hormel*	2 patties	400	2 M, 6 F
Tripe, beef, *Armour*	6 oz.	310	3 M, 3 F
Turkey,			
Swanson, **boned**	2½ oz.	110	2 M
Tender Chunk	3 oz.	90	2 M

■ Frozen and Refrigerated

Chicken, *Perdue,* *			
White meat	3½ oz.	160	3 M
Dark meat	3½ oz.	190	2½ M, 1 F
Breast	1 breast (about 8½ oz. without fat, skin, or bone).	300	5½ M
Cornish game hen, *Perdue,* *			
White meat	3½ oz.	150	2½ M
Dark meat	3½ oz.	180	2½ M, 1 F
Ham,			
Hormel,			
Bone-in	6 oz.	310	4 M, 2 F
Cure 81	6 oz.	290	4½ M, 1 F
Curemaster	6 oz.	210	4 M
Oscar Mayer Jubilee,			
Boneless	3 oz.	150	2 M, ½ F
Slice	3 oz.	90	1½ M
Steaks, 95% fat-free	1 steak	60	1 M
Turkey, **			
Breast,			
Land O'Lakes	3 oz.	100	2 M
Louis Rich	3½ oz.	165	3 M
Slices, *Louis Rich*	3½ oz.	140	2½ M
Tenderloins, *Louis Rich*	3½ oz.	145	2½ M
Diced, white/dark, *Land O'Lakes*	3 oz.	120	2 M
Drumsticks,			
Land O' Lakes	3 oz.	120	2½ M
Louis Rich	3½ oz.	210	4 M
Smoked, *Louis Rich*	3½ oz.	150	3 M
Ground, *Louis Rich*	3½ oz.	225	3½ M, ½ F
Ham, *Land O'Lakes*	3 oz.	100	2 M

*Edible portion, including skin.
**Edible portion, cooked.

Product Name	Serving Size	Calories	Exchanges
Hindquarters roast, *Land O'Lakes*	3 oz.	140	2½ M
Patties, *Land O' Lakes*	2¼ oz.	170	½ B, 1 M, 2 F
Roast, *Land O' Lakes*			
White/dark with gravy	3 oz.	120	2 M
White with gravy	3 oz.	110	2 M
Roll, *Land O' Lakes*			
Mixed	3 oz.	110	2 M
White	3 oz.	110	2 M
Sticks, *Land O' Lakes*	2 sticks	150	½ B, 1 M, 1½ F
Thighs, *Land O' Lakes*	3 oz.	150	2½ M, ½ F
Wings,			
Land O' Lakes	3 oz.	120	2½ M
Louis Rich	3½ oz.	190	3½ M
Smoked Drummettes, *Louis Rich*	3½ oz.	160	3 M
Whole, *Land O' Lakes,*			
Self-basting	3 oz.	120	2 M
Young	3 oz.	130	2½ M
Young, butter-basted	3 oz.	140	2½ M

VEGETARIAN MEAT SUBSTITUTES

■ Canned

Bits,			
Loma Linda Tender Bits	4 pieces	74	1½ M
Worthington Veja-Bits	4.3 oz.	67	1 M
Burger,			
Loma Linda Redi-Burger	½-inch slice	120	2 M
Worthington Vegetarian Burger	⅓ cup	150	2 M, ½ B
"Chicken,"			
Loma Linda, fried, with gravy	2 pieces	190	½ B, 2 M, 1 F
Worthington Fri-Chik	1 piece	95	1 M, 2 F
"Chili," *Worthington*	½ cup	190	1 B, 1½ M, 1 F
Dinner cuts,			
Loma Linda 145, 150, or 151	2 cuts	110	2 M
Loma Linda 158	1 cut	60	1 M
"Franks," *Loma Linda,*			
Big Franks	1 frank	95	1½ M
Sizzle Franks	2 franks	160	1½ M, 1½ F
Dinner loaf, savory, *Loma Linda*	1 slice	140	1½ M, 1½ F

Product Name	Serving Size	Calories	Exchanges
Links,			
Loma Linda,			
Linketts	2 links	140	½ B, 2 M
Little Links	2 links	85	1 M, ½ F
Worthington,			
Saucettes	1 link	65	½ M, 1 F
Super-Links	1 link	120	1 M, 1 F
Veja-Links	1 link	65	½ M, 1 F
Luncheon "meat,"			
Loma Linda,			
Nuteena 090 or 095	½-inch slice	160	½ B, 1 M, 2 F
Nuteena 100	⅜-inch slice	180	½ B, 1 M, 2 F
Proteena	½-inch slice	140	2½ M
Vegelona	½-inch slice	95	2 M
Worthington, Numete	½-inch slice	160	½ B, 1 M, 1½ F
"Meatballs,"			
Loma Linda Tender Rounds with Gravy	3 meatballs	100	½ B, 1½ M
Worthington Non-Meat Balls	3 meatballs	120	½ B, ½ M, 1½ F
Sandwich spread, *Loma Linda*	3 tbsp.	69	½ M, ½ F
"Scallops,"			
Loma Linda Vege-Scallops	6 pieces	70	1½ M
Worthington Vegetable Scallops	½ cup	70	1½ M
"Steak," *Worthington,*			
Prime Stakes	1 piece with gravy	160	½ B, 1 M, 1½ F
Vegetable Steaks	2½ pieces	100	½ B, 1½ M
"Swiss Steak," with gravy, *Loma Linda*	1 steak	130	½ B, 1½ M, ½ F

■ Dry

Product Name	Serving Size	Calories	Exchanges
Burger,			
Loma Linda,			
Vege-Burger	½ cup	110	2 M
Vita-Burger	3 tbsp.	70	½ B, ½ M
Sahadi Vegetable Burger	1.3 oz. dry	120	½ B, 1½ M
Worthington Gran Burger	1 oz. dry	105	½ B, 1½ M
"Chicken," *Loma Linda Supreme*	¼ cup dry	50	1 M
"Fish," *Loma Linda Ocean Platter*	¼ cup dry	50	1 M
Patty mix, *Loma Linda*	1 patty	130	1½ M, 1 F
"Stew," *Loma Linda Stew Pac*	1 package	66	1 M

Product Name	Serving Size	Calories	Exchanges

■Frozen

"Beef," *Worthington,*

Diced	⅜ cup	90	1 M, ½ F
Roll	1½ slices	90	1 M, ½ F
Smoked	5 slices	85	1 M, ½ F

"Bologna,"

Loma Linda	2 slices	140	2 M, ½ F
Worthington Bolono	2 slices	70	1 M

Burger,

Loma Linda Sizzle Burger	1 burger	190	½ B, 2 M, 1 F
Worthington Fri Pats	1 patty	180	2 M, 1½ F

"Chicken,"

Loma Linda, **fried**	1 piece	140	1½ M, 1½ F

Worthington,

Chic-ketts	1 oz.	60	1 M
Chik Stiks	1 piece	120	1 M, 1 F
Diced	⅜ cup	105	1 M, 1 F
Roll	1½ slices	105	1 M, 1 F

"Chops," *Worthington Choplets*	1 piece	50	1 M
"Corned beef," *Worthington*	3 slices	120	1 M, 1 F
"Cutlets," *Worthington*	1½ slices	90	½ B, 1 M

"Fish,"

Loma Linda Ocean Filet	1 filet	180	½ B, 2 M, 1 F
Worthington Filet	2 pieces	230	1 B, 2 M, 1 F

"Franks," *Loma Linda Corn Dogs*	1 frank	200	1½ B, ½ M, 1½ F
"Ham," *Worthington Wham*	2 slices	94	1 M, ½ F
"Meatballs," *Loma Linda*	4 pieces	190	½ B, 3 M
Roast, dinner, *Worthington*	2 oz. (½-inch slice)	140	1 M, 1½ F

"Salami,"

Loma Linda	2 slices	120	2 M
Worthington	2 slices	100	1 M, ½ F

"Sausage," *Worthington Prosage,*

Links	2 links	120	1 M, 1 F
Patties	1 patty	100	1 M, ½ F
Roll	⅜-inch slice	85	1 M, ½ F

"Steak,"

Loma Linda Griddle Steaks	1 steak	160	1½ M, 1½ F
Worthington Stakelets	1 piece	180	1½ M, 1½ F, ½ B

"Tuna," *Worthington Tuno*	2 oz.	90	½ M, 1 F
"Turkey," **smoked,** *Worthington*	2 slices	100	1 M, 1 F

2

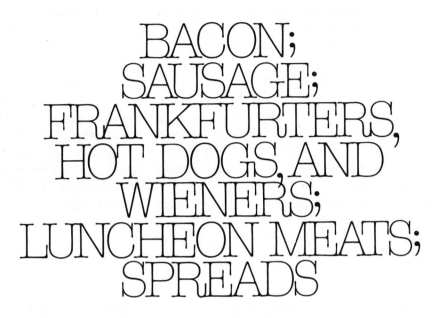

BACON;
SAUSAGE;
FRANKFURTERS,
HOT DOGS, AND
WIENERS;
LUNCHEON MEATS;
SPREADS

Processed meats listed here have been smoked, salted, or cured to improve flavor and keeping quality. All provide complete protein, but they tend to be high in sodium, saturated fat, and cholesterol. Frankfurters, wieners, and bologna, for example, can contain up to 30% fat. To reduce the fat content of your meal, choose turkey or chicken versions of these items with smaller amounts of fat, or luncheon meats like lean turkey and chicken breast and rolls, which are quite low in fat. Some companies also market reduced-fat luncheon meats, which are identified as such on the label.

Most items in this chapter fall into the "high-fat meat exchange" list of the ADA's

Exchange Lists for Meal Planning. However, here, as in the rest of this book, we give the exchanges in terms of lean meat exchanges plus fat exchanges, so that you can easily compare the items with other protein-rich foods such as fish, peas, beans, nuts, and other meats. When planning meals around protein-rich foods, it's helpful to compare the number of fat exchanges in a product with the number of meat exchanges. Here are some approximate guidelines:

Luncheon Meats One to two fat exchanges per meat exchange for most beef and pork items (bologna, salami, liverwurst).

	No fat exchanges for most turkey and chicken items.
Bacon	One to two fat exchanges per meat exchange for regular bacon. Imitation bacon products ("breakfast strips") are generally leaner (one fat exchange per meat exchange). Canadian-style bacon is quite lean (no fat exchanges).
Sausage	Two to three fat exchanges per meat exchange, except for turkey sausages (about one fat exchange per meat exchange).
Frankfurters, Hot Dogs, and Wieners	Up to three fat exchanges per meat exchange, except for turkey and chicken franks (about one fat exchange per meat exchange).

Remember, as always, to work *all* the exchanges into your meal plan. If the item is listed in ounces rather than per piece or per slice, use your food scale to measure portions accurately. Because fat is a concentrated source of calories (9 calories per gram), a small difference in weight for these high-fat items can mean a large difference in calories.

Product Name	Serving Size	Calories	Exchanges

BACON

Hormel,

Black Label	4 slices	140	1½ M, 1½ F
Range Brand	2 slices	90	1 M, 1 F
Red Label	4 slices	150	1 M, 2 F
Oscar Mayer,	2 slices	70	½ M, 1 F
Canadian-style, 93% fat-free	1 slice	40	1 M
Lean 'n Tasty Breakfast Strips,			
Beef	1 slice	40	½ M, ½ F
Pork	1 slice	40	½ M, ½ F
One-eighth-inch thick slices	2 slices	140	1 M, 2 F
Wafer thin	2 slices	80	½ M, 1 F

SAUSAGE

Banner, *Armour,*

10½ oz. pkg.	5.25 oz.	310	3 M, 3 F
24 oz. pkg.	4.0 oz.	240	2½ M, 2½ F
Breakfast, turkey, *Louis Rich*	1 oz. cooked	65	1 M
Hot, *Lance*	1 pkg. (0.75 oz.)	53	½ M, ½ F
Kielbasa, *Hormel Kolbase*	3 oz.	240	2 M, 3 F

Product Name	Serving Size	Calories	Exchanges

Pork,

Hormel,

Brown and Serve	4 sausages	310	2 M, 4½ F
Little Sizzlers	4 sausages	270	2 M, 3½ F
Midget Links	4 sausages	450	4 M, 5 F

Oscar Mayer,

Little Friers	1 link	80	½ M, 1 F
Southern Brand	1 patty	125	1 M, 1½ F

Smoked,

Hormel,

No-Link	3 oz.	290	2 M, 4 F
Smokies	4 sausages	370	2 M, 5½ F
Louis Rich, **turkey**	1 oz.	55	½ M, ½ F

Oscar Mayer,

Beef Smokies	1 link	130	1 M, 1½ F
Cheese Smokies	1 link	145	1 M, 2 F
Little Smokies	2 links	60	½ M, 1 F
Smokie Links	1 link	135	1 M, 2 F

FRANKFURTERS, HOT DOGS, AND WIENERS

Frankfurters,

Beef,

Oscar Mayer	1 frank	145	½ M, 2½ F
Oscar Mayer "The Big One"	1 frank	360	2 M, 5½ F
Oscar Mayer Jumbo	1 frank	185	1 M, 3 F
Chicken, Weaver	1 frank	120	1 M, 1½ F
Cocktail, Hebrew National	1 frank	48	1 F
Collagen, Hebrew National	1 frank	209	1 M, 3½ F
Natural casing, Hebrew National	1 frank	170	1 M, 2½ F
Skinless, Hebrew National	1 frank	160	1 M, 2½ F

Smoked, *Hormel*

Beef Wranglers	1 frank	160	1 M, 2½ F
Range Brand Wranglers	1 frank	180	1 M, 2½ F
Turkey, Louis Rich	1 frank	100	1 M, 1 F

Wieners,

Hormel,

Beef, 12 oz. pkg.	2 wieners	210	1½ M, 3 F
Beef, 16 oz. pkg.	1 wiener	140	1 M, 2 F
Batter-wrapped Corn Dogs	1 wiener	230	1½ B, ½ M, 2 F
Batter-wrapped Tater Dogs	1 wiener	190	1 B, ½ M, 2 F
Meat, 12 oz. pkg.	2 wieners	210	1 M, 3 F

Product Name	Serving Size	Calories	Exchanges
Meat, 16 oz. pkg.	1 wiener	140	1 M, 2 F
Oscar Mayer,	1 wiener	145	½ M, 2½ F
"The Big One"	1 wiener	365	2 M, 5½ F
with Cheese	1 wiener	145	½ M, 2½ F
Jumbo	1 wiener	185	1 M, 3 F
Little	2 wieners	60	½ M, 1 F

LUNCHEON MEATS *

Barb-B-Q loaf, 90% fat-free, Oscar Mayer	1 slice	50	½ M, ½ F
Beef,			
Chopped, Armour	3 oz.	290	1½ M, 4½ F
Dried sliced, Armour	1¼ oz.	60	1 M
Jerky, Lance,			
4.8 g pkg.	1 pkg.	18	½ M
7.3 g pkg.	1 pkg.	28	½ M
Smoked, Buddig	1 oz.	39	½ M
Snack, Lance,			
9.3 g pkg.	1 pkg.	53	½ M, ½ F
15.9 g pkg.	1 pkg.	90	½ M, 1½ F
Bologna,			
Oscar Mayer	1 slice	75	½ M, 1 F
Beef,	1 slice	75	½ M, 1 F
Oscar Mayer	1 slice	75	½ M, 1 F
Garlic, Oscar Mayer	1 slice	75	½ M, 1 F
Hickory-smoked, Fallowfield's	2 oz.	155	1½ M, 1 F
Lebanon, Oscar Mayer	1 slice	50	½ M, ½ F
Midget or sliced, Hebrew National	1 oz.	95	½ M, 1½ F
with Cheese, Oscar Mayer	1 slice	75	½ M, 1 F
Chicken, Weaver	1 oz.	80	½ M, 1 F
Coarse ground, Hormel	2 oz.	150	1 M, 2 F
Fine ground, Hormel	2 oz.	160	1 M, 2½ F
German, Oscar Mayer	1 slice	55	½ M, ½ F
Meat, Hormel	2 oz.	170	1 M, 2½ F
Ring, Oscar Mayer	1 oz.	80	½ M, 1 F
Turkey, Louis Rich	1 slice	60	½ M, ½ F
Braunschweiger, Oscar Mayer,			
German Brand	1 oz.	95	½ M, 1½ F
Liver sausage, sliced	1 slice	95	½ M, 1½ F

---

* One slice is equal to approximately one ounce.

Product Name	Serving Size	Calories	Exchanges
Liver sausage, tube	1 oz.	95	½ M, 1½ F
Chicken,			
Roll, white meat, *Weaver*	1 oz.	40	½ M
Smoked, *Buddig*	1 oz.	47	1 M
Corned beef,			
Brisket, cooked, *Hebrew National*	1 oz.	72	1 M, ½ F
Cooked, *Buddig*	1 oz.	39	½ M
Cooked and sliced, *Hebrew National*	1 oz.	64	1 M
Loaf, *Featherweight*	2½ oz.	90	1½ M
Jellied, 93% fat-free, *Oscar Mayer*	1 slice	40	1 M
Garlic ring, *Hebrew National*	1 oz.	90	½ M, 1½ F
Ham,			
and Cheese loaf, *Oscar Mayer*	1 slice	75	½ M, 1 F
Chopped,			
Armour	3 oz.	180	2 M, 1½ F
Hormel	1 oz.	70	1 M, ½ F
Oscar Mayer	1 slice	65	½ M, ½ F
Cooked,			
Hormel	2 oz.	70	1½ M
95% fat-free, *Oscar Mayer*	1 slice	25	½ M
Roll sausage, 92% fat-free, *Oscar Mayer*	1 slice	35	½ M
Smoked, *Buddig*	1 oz.	48	1 M
Head cheese, *Oscar Mayer*	1 slice	55	½ M, ½ F
Honey loaf, 95% fat-free, *Oscar Mayer*	1 slice	35	½ M
Honey roll sausage, 90% fat-free, *Oscar Mayer*	1 slice	40	½ M
Liver cheese, *Oscar Mayer*	1 slice	115	1 M, 1½ F
Liverwurst, *Hebrew National*	1 oz.	80	½ M, 1 F
Luncheon meat,			
Oscar Mayer	1 slice	100	½ M, 1½ F
Spam,	3 oz.	260	1½ M, 4 F
with Cheese chunks	3 oz.	260	1½ M, 4 F
Smoke flavored	3 oz.	260	1½ M, 4 F
Treet	3 oz.	300	1½ M, 4½ F
Spiced, *Hormel*	1 oz.	80	½ M, 1 F
Turkey, *Louis Rich*	1 slice	40	½ M, ½ F
Luxury loaf, 95% fat-free, *Oscar Mayer*	1 slice	40	½ M
Mortadella, *Oscar Mayer*	1 slice	50	1 F

Product Name	Serving Size	Calories	Exchanges
New England Brand sausage, Oscar Mayer	1 slice	35	½ M
Olive loaf, *Oscar Mayer*	1 slice	65	½ M, 1 F
Pastrami,			
Navel, *Hebrew National*	1 oz.	95	½ M, 1½ F
Sliced, *Hebrew National*	1 oz.	106	1 M, 1 F
Smoked, *Buddig*	1 oz.	39	½ M
Turkey, *Louis Rich*	1 slice	35	½ M
Pepperoni, *Hormel*	1 oz.	140	1 M, 2 F
Picnic loaf, *Oscar Mayer*	1 slice	65	½ M, 1 F
Potted meat,			
Armour,			
3 oz. pkg.	1.5 oz.	90	½ M, 1½ F
5½ oz. pkg.	1.83 oz.	110	1 M, 1 F
Libby's	1.8 oz.	100	1 M, 1 F
Salami,			
Beef, midget or sliced, *Hebrew National*	1 oz.	90	½ M, 1½ F
for Beer, *Oscar Mayer*	1 slice	55	½ M, ½ F
Beef	1 slice	75	½ M, 1 F
Cotto,			
Oscar Mayer	1 slice	50	½ M, ½ F
Beef, *Oscar Mayer*	1 slice	50	½ M, ½ F
Turkey, *Louis Rich*	1 slice	50	½ M, ½ F
Dairy hard, *Hormel*	1 oz.	120	1 M, 1½ F
Genoa,			
Di Lusso	1 oz.	130	1 M, 1½ F
Oscar Mayer	2 slices	70	½ M, 1 F
Hard, *Oscar Mayer*	2 slices	70	½ M, 1 F
Summer sausage,			
Thuringer Cervelat,			
Oscar Mayer	1 slice	75	½ M, 1 F
Beef, *Oscar Mayer*	1 slice	75	½ M, 1 F
Turkey, *Louis Rich*	1 slice	50	½ M, ½ F
Thuringer, *Old Smokehouse*	1 oz.	100	1 M, 1 F
Tongue,			
Armour	3 oz.	190	2 M, 1½ F
Hebrew National	1 oz.	72	½ M, 1 F
Turkey,			
Breast,			
Barbecued, *Louis Rich*	1 oz.	40	1 M
Oven-cooked, *Land O' Lakes* Bronze **or** *Silver Label*	3 oz.	100	2 M

Product Name	Serving Size	Calories	Exchanges
Oven-cooked, *Land O' Lakes Gold Label*	3 oz.	120	2 M
Oven-roasted, *Louis Rich*	1 slice	30	½ M
Roll, *Weaver*	1 oz.	25	½ M
Smoked, *Louis Rich*	1 slice	20	½ M
Ham,			
Louis Rich	1 slice	35	½ M
Weaver	1 oz.	35	½ M
Chopped and formed, *Louis Rich*	1 slice	45	1 M
Smoked, *Buddig*	1 oz.	42	1 M
Smoked,			
Buddig	1 oz.	45	1 M
Louis Rich	1 slice	30	½ M
Vienna sausage,			
Hormel	4 sausages	210	1 M, 3 F
in Barbecue sauce,			
Armour	2.5 oz.	190	1 M, 3 F
Libby's	2½ oz.	180	1 M, 2½ F
in Beef broth, *Libby's*	2 oz.	160	1 M, 2½ F
in Beef stock, *Armour*	2 oz.	140	½ M, 2½ F
Smoked, *Armour*	2 oz.	180	1 M, 2½ F

SPREADS

Product Name	Serving Size	Calories	Exchanges
Cheese,			
and Bacon, *Oscar Mayer*	1 oz.	70	½ M, 1 F
and Salami, *Oscar Mayer*	1 oz.	65	½ M, 1 F
Chicken,			
Salad, *Carnation Sandwich Spread*	1.9 oz.	119	1 M, 1 F
Spread,			
Swanson	1 oz.	60	½ M, ½ F
Underwood, **Chunky**	2.4 oz.	150	1½ M, 1½ F
Corned beef, *Underwood*	2¼ oz.	120	1 M, 1½ F
Deviled ham,			
Armour	1.5 oz.	110	1 M, 1 F
Hormel	1 oz.	70	½ M, 1 F
Libby's	1½ oz.	130	1 M, 1½ F
Underwood	2¼ oz.	220	1 M, 3½ F
Deviled luncheon meat,			
Spam	1 oz.	80	½ M, 1 F
Treet	1.5 oz.	120	1 M, 1½ F

Product Name	Serving Size	Calories	Exchanges

Ham,

and Cheese spread, *Oscar Mayer* . . 1 oz. . . . . 70 . . . . ½ M, 1 F

Salad,

Carnation Sandwich Spread . . . . 1.9 oz. . . . . 107 . . . . 1 M, 1 F

Oscar Mayer . . . . 1 oz. . . . . 60 . . . . ½ M, ½ F

Liver pate, *Sell's* . . . . 2.4 oz. . . . . 220 . . . . 1½ M, 3 F

Liverwurst, *Underwood* . . . . 2.4 oz. . . . . 220 . . . . 1½ M, 3 F

Roast beef, *Underwood* . . . . 2.4 oz. . . . . 140 . . . . 1½ M, 1½ F

Sandwich, *Oscar Mayer* . . . . 1 oz. . . . . 65 . . . . ½ M, 1 F

Tuna salad, *Carnation*
Sandwich Spread . . . . 1.9 oz. . . . . 98 . . . . 1 M, 1 F

Turkey salad, *Carnation*
Sandwich Spread . . . . 1.9 oz. . . . . 109 . . . . 1 M, 1 F

3

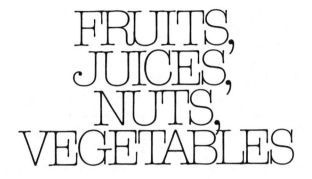

FRUITS, JUICES, NUTS, VEGETABLES

☐ Canned, dried, and frozen fruit

☐ Canned and ready-to-serve fruit and vegetable juices

☐ Nuts, nut butters, and seeds

☐ Canned and frozen vegetables and dry vegetable mixes

Fruits—dried, frozen, or canned in unsweetened juice or water—are a good source of vitamins (particularly A and C), minerals (particularly potassium), and fiber. Fruit's sweetness comes from *fructose*, a natural sugar that raises blood sugar only moderately. Fruit's natural fiber, or pulp, seems to slow the absorption of fruit sugar into the bloodstream, making fruit for dessert a healthy way to end a meal and satisfy a craving for sweets.

For your convenience, we've listed dried fruits, frozen fruits, and fruits canned in juice or water separately. Fruits canned in syrup have not been included, since they are high in calories and contain too much sugar. Many items listed here will exceed your allowed fruit exchanges if used as the manufacturer suggests, so reduce the serving size appropriately. Be especially careful with dried fruits, which are very concentrated—the manufacturer's recommended serving size may equal three or four fruit exchanges.

Pure fruit juices are also counted as fruit exchanges. Again, if the amount shown here exceeds your allowed exchanges, adjust the serving size accordingly. Although juices lack much of the fiber found in whole fruit, they too have vitamins and minerals and natural sweetness from fructose. (This is not true, however, of *juice drinks,* which may contain as little as 30% fruit juice, and *fruit-flavored drinks,* which may contain no juice at all. Because these items have usually been sweetened by sucrose or corn sweeteners, they should be avoided.) Because the sugar in fruit juice is absorbed rapidly, juices are useful for avoiding or counteracting insulin reactions. However, this rapid absorption, possibly caused by the absence of fruit fiber, may cause blood sugar levels to peak undesirably. You may want to consult your physician about this.

Vegetables and vegetable juices are also excellent sources of vitamins, minerals, and fiber. Nonstarchy vegetables (classified as vegetable exchanges) are low in calories. Starchy vegetables (classified as bread exchanges) rank higher in calories, but are good sources of complex carbohydrate. Particularly recommended are legumes such as peas, beans, and lentils. These items are high in protein and fiber as well as complex carbohydrate, and increase blood sugar only very moderately—less than most other bread exchange foods.*

Many items listed are combinations of exchanges—bread and vegetable exchanges for mixed vegetables containing both starchy and nonstarchy vegetables; vegetable and fat exchanges for nonstarchy vegetables in butter or sauce; and bread, vegetable, and fat exchanges for mixed vegetables in sauces or pastries. Serving sizes for many frozen vegetables are often given in ounces rather than in more common household measurements. However, you'll find that these portions correspond to some fraction of the package weight (usually ½, ⅓, or ¼). You needn't weigh your portion to get the correct exchange—simply divide the total package contents by the appropriate number (2, 3, or 4 for the examples above). Canned and frozen vegetables are listed separately, and there's an additional list of dried potato mixes.

Nuts and nut butters provide a concentrated source of protein, fat, and calories, as well as some B vitamins, vitamin E, magnesium, and zinc. They also contain some carbohydrate, but are classified on many exchange lists under their predominant component: fat. Here, we calculate them as a combination of meat and fat exchanges, which more accurately reflects their nutrient content. Bread exchanges were used to account for carbohydrate when present in 5 or more grams per serving. However, vegetarians who consume more than ¼ cup of nuts or seeds per day must account for the extra carbohydrate in *all* nuts and should talk to their dietitians about adjusting the number of allowed bread exchanges.

FRUIT

■ Canned

Applesauce,
  Del Monte . . . . ½ cup . . . . 90 . . . . 2½ Fr

---

*Jenkins, D., Wolever, T., Taylor, R., *et al. Am. J. Clin. Nutr.* 34:362, 1981.

Product Name	Serving Size	Calories	Exchanges
Featherweight water pack	½ cup	50	1 Fr
Apricot halves,			
Del Monte Lite	½ cup	60	1½ Fr
Featherweight,			
Juice pack	½ cup	50	1 Fr
Water pack	½ cup	35	1 Fr
Cherries,			
Dark sweet pitted, *Featherweight* water pack	½ cup	60	1½ Fr
Light sweet pitted, *Featherweight* water pack	½ cup	50	1 Fr
Fruit cocktail,			
Del Monte Lite	½ cup	50	1 Fr
Featherweight,			
Juice pack	½ cup	50	1 Fr
Water pack	½ cup	40	1 Fr
Weight Watchers	½ cup	60	1½ Fr
Fruit compote, *Rokeach*	4 oz.	120	3 Fr
Grapefruit, *Featherweight* juice pack	½ cup	40	1 Fr
Mandarin oranges, *Featherweight* water pack	½ cup	35	1 Fr
Mixed fruit, chunky, *Del Monte Lite*	½ cup	50	1 Fr
Peaches,			
Weight Watchers	½ cup	60	1½ Fr
Yellow cling,			
Del Monte Lite	½ cup	50	1 Fr
Featherweight juice pack	½ cup	50	1 Fr
Featherweight water pack	½ cup	30	1 Fr
Yellow freestone, *Featherweight* juice pack	½ cup	50	1 Fr
Pears,			
Featherweight juice pack	½ cup	60	1½ Fr
Weight Watchers	½ cup	60	1½ Fr
Bartlett,			
Del Monte Lite	½ cup	50	1 Fr
Featherweight water pack	½ cup	40	1 Fr
Pineapple,			
in Juice,			
Del Monte	½ cup	70	2 Fr
Dole	½ cup	70	2 Fr
Featherweight juice pack	½ cup	70	2 Fr

Product Name	Serving Size	Calories	Exchanges
in Water,			
Featherweight water pack	½ cup	60	1½ Fr
Plums, whole purple, *Featherweight,*			
Juice pack	½ cup	80	2 Fr
Water pack	½ cup	40	1 Fr
Prunes, stewed,			
Featherweight water pack	½ cup	130	3½ Fr

■Dried

Product Name	Serving Size	Calories	Exchanges
Apple,			
Chunks, *Sunsweet*	2 oz.	150	4 Fr
Sliced, *Del Monte*	2 oz.	140	3½ Fr
Apricots,			
Del Monte	2 oz.	140	3½ Fr
Sunsweet	2 oz.	140	3½ Fr
Currants, zante, *Del Monte*	½ cup	200	5 Fr
Dates, *Dromedary,*			
Chopped	1 tbsp.	33	1 Fr
Pitted	2 dates	40	1 Fr
Fig pieces, *Sun-Maid Mission Figlets*	½ cup	210	5½ Fr
Fruit bits, *Sun-Maid*	¾ oz.	70	2 Fr
Mixed fruit,			
Cookman's Preservative-Free	2 oz.	140	4 Fr
Del Monte	2 oz.	130	3½ Fr
Sunsweet	2 oz.	150	4 Fr
Peaches,			
Del Monte	2 oz.	140	3½ Fr
Sunsweet	2 oz.	140	3½ Fr
Prunes,			
Del Monte Moist-Pak	2 oz.	120	3 Fr
Sunsweet RTS	½ cup	120	3 Fr
Pitted,			
Del Monte	2 oz.	140	3½ Fr
Sunsweet	2 oz.	140	3½ Fr
with Pits, *Del Monte*	2 oz.	120	3 Fr
Raisins, *Sun-Maid*	½ cup	290	7 Fr

■Frozen

Product Name	Serving Size	Calories	Exchanges
Mixed, *Birds Eye Quick Thaw*	5 oz.	140	3½ Fr
Peaches, *Birds Eye Quick Thaw*	5 oz.	130	3½ Fr
Raspberries, Red,			
Birds Eye Quick Thaw	5 oz.	150	4 Fr

Product Name	Serving Size	Calories	Exchanges

Strawberries, *Birds Eye,*
   Quick Thaw . . . . 5 oz. . . . . 120 . . . . 3 Fr
   Whole . . . . 4 oz. . . . . 80 . . . . 2 Fr

FRUIT AND VEGETABLE JUICES

■ Frozen

Apple,
   Minute Maid . . . . 6 fl. oz. . . . . 100 . . . . 2½ Fr
   Seneca . . . . 6 fl. oz. . . . . 90 . . . . 2½ Fr
     Natural Style . . . . 6 fl. oz . . . . 90 . . . . 2½ Fr
   Tropicana . . . . 6 fl. oz. . . . . 83 . . . . 2 Fr
Cranberry apple, *Welch's* . . . . 6 fl. oz. . . . . 120 . . . . 3 Fr
Cranberry grape, *Welch's* . . . . 6 fl. oz. . . . . 110 . . . . 2½ Fr
Cranberry juice cocktail, *Welch's* . . . . 6 fl. oz. . . . . 100 . . . . 2½ Fr
Citrus, *Minute Maid Five Alive* . . . . . 6 fl. oz. . . . . 85 . . . . 2 Fr
Fruit punch,
   Minute Maid Five Alive . . . . 6 fl. oz. . . . . 87 . . . . 2 Fr
Grape, *Seneca* . . . . 6 fl. oz. . . . . 115 . . . . 3 Fr
Grapefruit,
   Minute Maid . . . . 6 fl. oz. . . . . 75 . . . . 2 Fr
   Tropicana . . . . 6 fl. oz. . . . . 76 . . . . 2 Fr
Lemon, *Minute Maid* . . . . 6 fl. oz. . . . . 40 . . . . 1 Fr
Lemonade, *Minute Maid* . . . . 6 fl. oz. . . . . 74 . . . . 2 Fr
Limeade, *Minute Maid* . . . . 6 fl. oz. . . . . 75 . . . . 2 Fr
Orange,
   Minute Maid, ... 6 fl. oz. . . . . 86 . . . . 2 Fr
     with More pulp . . . . 6 fl. oz. . . . . 86 . . . . 2 Fr
     Reduced acid . . . . 6 fl. oz. . . . . 86 . . . . 2 Fr
   Tropicana . . . . 6 fl. oz. . . . . 84 . . . . 2 Fr
   Imitation, *Bright and Early* . . . . 6 fl. oz. . . . . 90 . . . . 2½ Fr
Orange/grapefruit, *Minute Maid* . . . . 6 fl. oz. . . . . 76 . . . . 2 Fr
Pineapple, *Minute Maid* . . . . 6 fl. oz. . . . . 92 . . . . 2½ Fr
Pineapple/orange, *Minute Maid* . . . . 6 fl. oz. . . . . 94 . . . . 2½ Fr
Tangerine, *Minute Maid* . . . . 6 fl. oz. . . . . 85 . . . . 2 Fr

■ Ready to Serve (bottled and canned)

Apple,
   Minute Maid . . . . 6 fl. oz. . . . . 100 . . . . 2½ Fr
   Tropicana, **from concentrate** . . . . . 6 fl. oz. . . . . 83 . . . . 2 Fr
Apple/grape, *Weight Watchers* . . . . . ⅓ cup . . . . 45 . . . . 1 Fr

Product Name	Serving Size	Calories	Exchanges
Apricot nectar,			
Del Monte	6 fl. oz.	100	2½ Fr
Libby's	6 fl. oz.	110	2½ Fr
Banana nectar, *Libby's*	6 fl. oz.	60	1½ Fr
Cranberry juice cocktail,			
Ocean Spray	6 fl. oz.	110	2½ Fr
Cranberry/apple juice drink,			
Ocean Spray Cranapple	6 fl. oz.	130	3½ Fr
Low-calorie	6 fl. oz.	30	1 Fr
Cranberry/apricot juice drink,			
Ocean Spray Cranicot	6 fl. oz.	110	2½ Fr
Fruit Medley, *Weight Watchers*	⅓ cup	45	1 Fr
Fruit punch, *Minute Maid*	6 fl. oz.	93	2½ Fr
Grape,			
Welch's	6 fl. oz.	120	3 Fr
Red	6 fl. oz.	120	3 Fr
Sparkling red	6 fl. oz.	120	3 Fr
Sparkling white	6 fl. oz.	120	3 Fr
White	6 fl. oz.	120	3 Fr
Grape/cranberry drink,			
Ocean Spray Crangrape	6 fl. oz.	110	2½ Fr
Grapefruit,			
Del Monte, **unsweetened**	6 fl. oz.	70	2 Fr
Libby's, **unsweetened**	6 fl. oz.	75	2 Fr
Minute Maid	6 fl. oz.	75	2 Fr
Ocean Spray	6 fl. oz.	60	1½ Fr
Tropicana, **from concentrate**	6 fl. oz.	76	2 Fr
Cocktail, pink, *Ocean Spray*	6 fl. oz.	80	2 Fr
Guava nectar, *Libby's*	6 fl. oz.	70	2 Fr
Lemon, from concentrate,			
Realemon	2 tbsp.	6	free
Lemonade, *Minute Maid*	6 fl. oz.	79	2 Fr
Pink	6 fl. oz.	78	2 Fr
Lime, from concentrate, *Realime*	2 tbsp.	4	free
Mango nectar, *Libby's*	6 fl. oz.	60	1½ Fr
Orange,			
Del Monte, **unsweetened**	6 fl. oz.	80	2 Fr
Libby's, **unsweetened**	6 fl. oz.	90	2½ Fr
Minute Maid	6 fl. oz.	83	2 Fr
Tropicana, **from concentrate**	6 fl. oz.	84	2 Fr
Orange and grapefruit juice,			
Libby's, **unsweetened**	6 fl. oz.	80	2 Fr
Peach nectar, *Libby's*	6 fl. oz.	90	2½ Fr

Product Name	Serving Size	Calories	Exchanges
Pear nectar, *Libby's*	6 fl. oz.	100	2½ Fr
Pear/passion fruit nectar, *Libby's*	6 fl. oz.	60	1½ Fr
Pineapple,			
Del Monte, unsweetened	6 fl. oz.	100	2½ Fr
Dole	6 fl. oz.	103	2½ Fr
Prune,			
Del Monte, unsweetened	6 fl. oz.	120	3 Fr
Sunsweet	⅖ cup	75	2 Fr
Strawberry nectar, *Libby's*	6 fl. oz.	60	1½ Fr
Tomato,			
Campbell's	6 fl. oz.	35	1 V
Low sodium	6 fl. oz.	35	1 V
Featherweight	6 fl. oz.	35	1 V
Libby's	6 fl. oz.	35	1 V
Welch's	6 fl. oz.	35	1 V
Cocktail, *Snap-E-Tom*	6 fl. oz.	40	1½ V
Vegetable,			
Campbell's "V8,"	6 fl. oz.	35	1 V
Low-sodium	6 fl. oz.	35	1 V
Spicy hot	6 fl. oz.	40	1½ V
Featherweight	6 fl. oz.	35	1 V

NUTS, NUT BUTTERS, AND SEEDS

■ Nuts and Seeds

Product Name	Serving Size	Calories	Exchanges
Almonds,			
Fisher,			
Dry roasted	1 oz.	175	½ B, ½ M, 2½ F
Oil roasted	1 oz.	178	½ B, ½ M, 2½ F
Raw	1 oz.	170	½ B, ½ M, 2½ F
Lance	1 pkg. (⁹⁄₁₆ oz.)	100	½ M, 2 F
Cashews, *Fisher,*			
Dry roasted	1 oz.	156	½ B, ½ M, 2 F
Oil roasted	1 oz.	159	½ B, ½ M, 2 F
Filberts, *Fisher,* oil dipped	1 oz.	180	½ M, 3½ F
Nuts Galore, *Sun-Maid Nature Snacks*	1 oz.	170	1 M, 2½ F
Sunflower seeds, *Fisher,* roasted in shell	1 oz.	86	½ M, 1½ F
Peanuts,			
Fisher,			
Blanched, oil roasted	1 oz.	166	½ B, 1 M, 2 F

Product Name	Serving Size	Calories	Exchanges
Dry roasted	1 oz.	163	½ B, 1 M, 2 F
Redskin, oil roasted	1 oz.	165	½ B, 1 M, 2 F
Roasted in shell	1 oz.	105	½ M, 2 F
Lance,			
Redskins	1 pkg. (1¼ oz.)	216	1½ M, 3 F
Roasted in shell	1 pkg. (1¾ oz.)	185	1½ M, 2½ F
Salted	1 pkg. (1⅛ oz.)	192	1½ M, 2½ F
Peanuts and raisins, dry roasted, *Fisher*	1 oz.	130	½ B, ½ M, 1 F, ½ Fr
Pecans, *Fisher,*			
Oil dipped	1 oz.	195	½ M, 4 F
Raw	1 oz.	195	½ M, 4 F
Pistachios, roasted in shell, *Fisher*	1 oz.	84	½ M, 1½ F
Walnuts,			
Diamond	¼ cup	340	1½ M, 5½ F
Fisher,			
Black, raw	1 oz.	178	½ M, 3½ F
English, raw	1 oz.	185	½ M, 3½ F

■ Nut Butters

Peanut butter,			
Bama,			
Creamy	2 tbsp.	200	1 M, 3 F
Crunchy	2 tbsp.	200	1 M, 3 F
Dia-Mel	2 tbsp.	200	1 M, 3 F
Featherweight low sodium	2 tbsp.	180	1 M, 2½ F
Peter Pan,			
Creamy	2 tbsp.	190	1 M, 3 F
Crunchy	2 tbsp.	190	1 M, 3 F
Low sodium	2 tbsp.	190	1 M, 3 F
Skippy	2 tbsp.	190	1 M, 3 F
Smucker's,			
Natural	2 tbsp.	200	1 M, 3 F
No salt added	2 tbsp.	200	1 M, 3 F
Sesame tahini, *Sahadi*	2 tbsp.	190	1 M, 3 F

VEGETABLES

■ Canned

Asparagus,			
Del Monte	½ cup	20	1 V

Product Name	Serving Size	Calories	Exchanges
Green Giant	½ cup	25	1 V
Bamboo shoots, *La Choy*	¼ cup drained	6	free in moderation
Bean sprouts, *La Choy*	⅔ cup drained	8	free in moderation
Beans,			
and Bacon, *Hormel Short Orders*	7½ oz.	340	2½ B, 1½ M, 2 F
Baked,			
Red kidney, *B&M*	⅞ cup	330	3½ B, 1 M, 1 F
Red kidney, *Friend's*	1 cup	340	4 B, 1½ M
Small pea, *B&M*	⅞ cup	330	3½ B, 1 M, 1 F
Small pea, *Friend's*	1 cup	360	4 B, 1½ M
Yellow eye, *B&M*	⅞ cup	330	3½ B, 1 M, 1 F
Yellow eye, *Friend's*	1 cup	360	4 B, 1½ M
Barbeque, *Campbell's*	4 oz.	125	1½ B, ½ F
Burrito filling, *Del Monte*	½ cup	110	1 B, ½ M
Butter, *Van Camp*	8 oz.	160	2 B, ½ M
and Franks in tomato and molasses sauce, *Campbell's*	4 oz.	175	1½ B, ½ M, 1 F
and Franks in tomato sauce, *Heinz*	7¾ oz.	330	2 B, 1 M, 1 V, 2 F
and Ham, *Hormel Short Orders*	7½ oz.	370	2½ B, 1½ M, 2½ F
Homestyle, *Campbell's*	4 oz.	135	1½ B, ½ F
Kidney, *Van Camp,*			
Dark red	8 oz.	180	2½ B, ½ M
Light red	8 oz.	180	2½ B, ½ M
New Orleans style	8 oz.	180	2½ B, ½ M
Mexican-style chili, *Van Camp*	8 oz.	210	2½ B, 1 M
Old fashioned in molasses and brown sugar sauce, *Campbell's*	4 oz.	135	1½ B, ½ F
and Pork,			
Van Camp	8 oz.	220	2½ B, 1 M
in Tomato sauce, *Campbell's*	4 oz.	125	1½ B, ½ F
in Tomato sauce, *Heinz*	8 oz.	250	2½ B, 1 M, 1 V
Red, *Van Camp*	8 oz.	190	2½ B, ½ M
Refried,			
Del Monte	½ cup	130	1½ B, ½ M
Old El Paso	½ cup	100	1 B, ½ M
with Green chilies, *Old El Paso*	½ cup	92	1 B, ½ M
with Sausage, *Old El Paso*	½ cup	194	1 B, ½ M, 2 F
Spicy, *Del Monte*	½ cup	130	1½ B, ½ M
in Tomato sauce, vegetarian, *Heinz*	8 oz.	230	2½ B, ½ M, 1 V
Vegetarian style, *Van Camp*	8 oz.	210	2½ B, 1 M

Product Name	Serving Size	Calories	Exchanges
Western style, *Van Camp*	8 oz.	210	2½ B, 1 M
and Wieners,			
Hormel Short Orders	7½ oz.	290	2 B, 1 M, 2 F
Van Camp Beanee Weenee	8 oz.	300	2 B, 1½ M, 2 F
Beets,			
Del Monte	½ cup	35	1 V
Featherweight	½ cup	45	1½ V
Carrots, sliced, *Featherweight*	½ cup	30	1 V
Chop suey vegetables, *La Choy*	½ cup drained	10	½ V
Corn,			
Whole kernel,			
Del Monte	½ cup	70	1 B
Del Monte **vacuum-packed**	½ cup	90	1½ B
Del Monte **white**	½ cup	70	1 B
Featherweight	½ cup	80	1 B
Green Giant	½ cup	80	1 B
Green Giant **golden and white shoe peg**	½ cup	90	1½ B
Green Giant **vacuum-packed**	½ cup	90	1½ B
Green Giant Mexicorn	½ cup	100	1½ B
Cream style,			
Del Monte	½ cup	80	1 B
Del Monte white	½ cup	90	1½ B
Green beans,			
Del Monte **cut, French style, or whole**	½ cup	20	1 V
Featherweight	½ cup	25	1 V
Italian, *Del Monte*	½ cup	25	1 V
Lima beans,			
Del Monte	½ cup	70	1 B
Featherweight	½ cup	80	1 B
Mixed vegetables,			
Del Monte	½ cup	40	½ B
Featherweight	½ cup	40	½ B
Chinese, *La Choy*	½ cup drained	12	½ V
Mushrooms, *Green Giant*	2 oz.	14	½ V
Onions,			
Boiled, *O&C*	2 oz.	16	½ V
French fried, *Durkee*	1 oz.	178	½ B, 3 F
Peas,			
Del Monte,			
Small sweet	½ cup	50	1 B

Product Name	Serving Size	Calories	Exchanges
Sweet	½ cup	60	1 B
Featherweight	½ cup	70	1 B
Green Giant,			
Early June	½ cup	60	1 B
Minisweet	½ cup	60	1 B
Sweet	½ cup	60	1 B
and Carrots, *Del Monte*	½ cup	50	½ B, ½ V
and Onions, *Green Giant*	½ cup	60	½ B, ½ V
Seasoned, *Del Monte*	½ cup	60	1 B
Pimientos, *Del Monte,* diced, sliced, or whole	2 tbsp.	8	free in moderation
Potatoes, *Del Monte,* sliced or whole	½ cup	45	½ B
Pumpkin,			
Del Monte	1 cup	70	1 B
Libby's solid pack	1 cup	80	1 B
Sauerkraut, *Del Monte*	½ cup	25	1 V
Spinach, *Del Monte,* chopped or whole leaf	½ cup	25	1 V
Three-bean salad, *Green Giant*	½ cup	90	1 B, ½ V
Tomatoes,			
Contadina,			
Baby sliced	½ cup	50	1½ V
Italian-style pear	½ cup	25	1 V
Stewed	½ cup	35	1 V
Whole peeled	½ cup	25	1 V
Del Monte,			
Stewed	½ cup	35	1 V
Wedges	½ cup	30	1 V
Whole peeled	½ cup	25	1 V
Featherweight	½ cup	20	1 V
and Green chilies, *Old El Paso*	3½ oz.	23	1 V
and Jalapenos, *Ortega*	1 oz.	7	free in moderation
Tomato paste,			
Contadina	¼ cup	50	½ B, 1 V
Italian	¼ cup	70	½ B, 1 V
Italian with mushrooms	¼ cup	60	½ B, 1 V
Cookman's Preservative-Free	¼ cup	55	½ B, 1 V
Del Monte	¾ cup	150	1½ B, 1½ V
Featherweight	6 oz.	150	1½ B, 1½ V
Tomato purée,			
Contadina	½ cup	50	½ B, 1 V

Product Name	Serving Size	Calories	Exchanges
Featherweight	1 cup	90	1 B, 1 V
Tomato sauce,			
Contadina	½ cup	45	½ B, ½ V
Italian style	½ cup	40	½ B, ½ V
Del Monte	1 cup	70	½ B, 1½ V
with Onions	1 cup	100	1 B, 1 V
Water chestnuts, *La Choy*	¼ cup drained and sliced	16	½ V
Wax beans,			
Del Monte	½ cup	20	1 V
Featherweight	½ cup	25	1 V

■ Frozen

Product Name	Serving Size	Calories	Exchanges
Artichoke hearts, *Birds Eye*	3 oz.	30	1 V
Asparagus,			
Birds Eye,			
Cut	3.3 oz.	25	1 V
Jumbo spears	3.3 oz.	25	1 V
Spears	3.3 oz.	25	1 V
in Butter sauce, *Green Giant*	½ cup	70	1 V, 1 F
with Mornay sauce in pastry, *Pepperidge Farm*	1 piece	250	1 B, 1 V, 3½ F
Soufflé, *Stouffer's*	4.0 oz.	115	½ V, 1½ F, ½ Mk
Black-eye peas, *Birds Eye*	3.3 oz.	130	1½ B, 1 M
Broccoli,			
Birds Eye,			
Chopped	3.3 oz.	25	1 V
Cuts	3.3 oz.	25	1 V
Florets	3.3 oz.	25	1 V
Spears	3.3 oz.	25	1 V
Spears, baby	3.3 oz.	30	1 V
Harvest Fresh cuts and spears	½ cup	30	1 V
with Almonds, *Birds Eye*	3.3 oz.	60	1 V, ½ F
Baby carrots, and water chestnuts, *Birds Eye*	3.2 oz.	30	1 V
in Butter sauce, *Green Giant*	½ cup	40	½ B, ½ V
Carrots, and pasta twists, *Birds Eye*	3.3 oz.	90	½ B, 1 V, ½ F
Cauliflower, and carrots, *Birds Eye*	3.2 oz.	25	1 V
Cauliflower, and carrots with cheese sauce, *Birds Eye*	5 oz.	130	½ B, 1 V, 1½ F

Product Name	Serving Size	Calories	Exchanges
Green Giant	½ cup	60	½ B, ½ V, ½ F
Cauliflower, corn, and pasta, *Birds Eye*	3.3 oz.	110	½ B, 1 V, 1 F
Cauliflower medley, *Harvest Get Together*	½ cup	60	2 V
Cauliflower, and red peppers, *Birds Eye*	3.3 oz.	25	1 V
with Cheese sauce,			
Birds Eye	5 oz.	170	½ B, 1 V, 2½ F
Green Giant	½ cup	70	½ B, ½ V, ½ F
Stouffer's	4½ oz.	130	1 M, 1 V, 1 F
White cheddar, *Green Giant*	½ cup	70	½ B, ½ V, ½ F
and Cheese, light batter, *Mrs. Paul's*	2½ oz.	150	½ M, ½ B, 1 V, 1½ F
with Cheese in pastry, *Pepperidge Farm*	1 piece	250	1 B, 1 V, 3½ F
Corn, and red peppers, *Birds Eye*	3.2 oz.	50	½ B, ½ V
Fanfare, *Harvest Get Together*	½ cup	80	½ B, 1 V, ½ F
Green beans, onions, and red peppers, *Birds Eye*	3.2 oz.	25	1 V
Pasta, onions, and mushrooms, *Birds Eye*	3.3 oz.	100	½ B, ½ V, 1 F
with Water chestnuts, *Birds Eye*	3.3 oz.	35	1 V
Brussels sprouts,			
Birds Eye	3.3 oz.	35	1 V
Baby	3.3 oz.	40	1½ V
in Butter sauce, *Green Giant*	½ cup	60	½ B, ½ V, ½ F
Cauliflower, and carrots, *Birds Eye*	3.2 oz.	30	1 V
in Cheese sauce,			
Green Giant	½ cup	80	½ B, ½ V, ½ F
Baby, *Birds Eye*	4.5 oz.	150	½ B, 1 V, 2 F
Butter beans, baby, *Birds Eye*	3.3 oz.	140	1½ B, ½ M
Cantonese-Style Stir Fry, *Birds Eye*	3.3 oz.	50	½ B, 1 V
Cabbage pierogies, *Mrs. Paul's*	5 oz.	330	4 B, ½ V, 1 F
Carrots,			
Birds Eye, **whole baby**	3.3 oz.	40	1½ V
in Butter sauce, *Green Giant*	½ cup	80	½ B, ½ V, ½ F
Sweet peas, and pearl onions, *Birds Eye*	3.3 oz.	50	½ B, ½ V
Cauliflower,			
Birds Eye,	3.3 oz.	25	1 V
Florets	3.3 oz.	25	1 V
with Almonds, *Birds Eye*	3.3 oz.	40	1 V, ½ F

Product Name	Serving Size	Calories	Exchanges
Carrot Bonanza,			
Harvest Get Together	½ cup	60	½ B, ½ V, ½ F
and Cheese, light batter,			
Mrs. Paul's	2.6 oz.	120	1 B, ½ V, 1 F
with Cheese sauce,			
Birds Eye	5.0 oz.	160	½ B, 1 V, 2 F
Green Giant	½ cup	60	½ B, ½ V, ½ F
White cheddar, *Green Giant*	½ cup	70	½ B, ½ V, ½ F
in Pastry, *Pepperidge Farm*	1 piece	220	1 B, 1 V, 2½ F
Green beans, and corn, *Birds Eye*	3.2 oz.	35	½ B, ½ V
Chinese Style,			
Oriental Combination	½ cup	60	1 V, ½ F
with Seasoned sauce, *Birds Eye*	3.3 oz.	25	1 V
Stir Fry, *Birds Eye*	3.3 oz.	30	1 V
Collard greens, chopped, *Birds Eye*	3.3 oz.	25	1 V
Corn,			
Birds Eye sweet whole kernel	3.3 oz.	80	1 B
Harvest Fresh	½ cup	100	1½ B
in Butter sauce,			
Green Giant Niblets	½ cup	100	1 B, ½ F
Green Giant white shoe peg	½ cup	100	1 B, ½ F
on the Cob, *Birds Eye Little Ears*	2 ears	130	2 B
in Cream sauce, *Green Giant*	½ cup	130	1½ B, ½ F
Fritters, *Mrs. Paul's*	4 oz.	260	2½ B, 2 F
Green beans, and pasta curls, *Birds Eye*	3.3 oz.	110	1 B, 1 F
Soufflé, *Stouffer's*	4 oz.	155	1 B, 1 F, ½ Mk
Eggplant,			
Parmesan, *Mrs. Paul's*	5½ oz.	250	1 B, ½ M, 1 V, 3 F
Sticks, *Mrs. Paul's*	3½ oz.	260	1½ B, 1 V, 3 F
Green beans,			
Birds Eye,			
Cut	3.0 oz.	25	1 V
French style	3.0 oz.	25	1 V
Whole	3.0 oz.	25	1 V
Harvest Fresh	½ cup	25	1 V
Bavarian style, and spaetzle, with seasoned sauce, *Birds Eye*	3.3 oz.	50	½ B, 1 V
in Butter sauce, *Green Giant*	½ cup	35	1 V, ½ F
Cauliflower, and carrots, *Birds Eye*	3.2 oz.	25	1 V
Corn, carrots and pearl onions, *Birds Eye*	3.2 oz.	40	½ B, ½ V

Product Name	Serving Size	Calories	Exchanges
in Cream sauce, *Green Giant*	½ cup	80	½ B, ½ V, ½ F
Italian, *Birds Eye*	3.0 oz.	30	1 V
Mushroom casserole, *Stouffer's*	4¾ oz.	150	½ B, 1 V, 2 F
with Sliced mushrooms, *Birds Eye*	3.0 oz.	30	1 V
with Toasted almonds, *Birds Eye*	3.0 oz.	50	1 V, ½ F
Italian Style with seasoned sauce, *Birds Eye*	3.3 oz.	60	½ B, ½ V, ½ F
Japanese Style,			
Oriental Combination	½ cup	45	½ B, ½ V
with Seasoned sauce, *Birds Eye*	3.3 oz.	40	½ B, ½ V
Stir Fry, *Birds Eye*	3.3 oz.	30	1 V
Kale, chopped, *Birds Eye*	3.3 oz.	25	1 V
Lima beans,			
Birds Eye,			
Baby	3.3 oz.	130	1½ B, ½ M
Fordhook	3.3 oz.	100	1 B, ½ M
Tiny	3.3 oz.	110	1 B, ½ M
Harvest Fresh	½ cup	100	1 B, ½ M
in Butter sauce, *Green Giant*	½ cup	120	1½ B, ½ F
Mixed vegetables,			
Birds Eye	3.3 oz.	60	½ B, ½ V
Harvest Fresh	½ cup	60	½ B, ½ V
in Butter sauce, *Green Giant*	½ cup	60	½ B, ½ V, ½ F
with Onion sauce, *Birds Eye*	2.6 oz.	110	½ B, ½ V, 1 F
Mushrooms,			
in Butter sauce, *Green Giant*	½ cup	70	1 V, 1 F
Dijon, in pastry, *Pepperidge Farm*	1 piece	230	1 B, 1 V, 3 F
Mustard greens, chopped, *Birds Eye*	3.3 oz.	20	1 V
New England Style with seasoned sauce, *Birds Eye*	3.3 oz.	70	½ B, 1 V
Okra, *Birds Eye,*			
Cut	3.3 oz.	25	1 V
Whole	3.3 oz.	30	1 V
Onions,			
Birds Eye,			
Chopped	2 oz.	16	½ V
Pearl	3.3 oz.	35	1 V
Small whole	4 oz.	40	1½ V
Rings, fried, *Mrs. Paul's*	2½ oz.	150	1 B, 1 V, 1½ F
Small,			
in Cheese-flavored sauce, *Green Giant*	½ cup	90	½ B, ½ V, 1 F

Product Name	Serving Size	Calories	Exchanges
with Cream sauce, *Birds Eye*	3.0 oz.	100	½ B, ½ V, 1 F
Peas,			
Birds Eye,			
Sweet green	3.3 oz.	80	1 B
Tiny tender	3.3 oz.	60	1 B
Harvest Fresh	½ cup	80	1 B
in Butter sauce, *Green Giant*	½ cup	90	1 B, ½ F
and Carrots, *Birds Eye*	3.3 oz.	60	½ B, ½ V
Carrots, pasta, and pearl onions, *Birds Eye*	3.3 oz.	120	1 B, ½ V, 1 F
Carrots, and pearl onions, *Birds Eye*	3.2 oz.	50	½ B, ½ V
with Cream sauce,			
Birds Eye	2.6 oz.	130	1 B, 1½ F
Green Giant	½ cup	100	½ B, ½ V, 1 F
Onions, and carrots in butter sauce, *Green Giant*	½ cup	90	½ B, ½ V, 1 F
Pea pods, and water chestnuts in butter sauce, *Green Giant*	½ cup	80	2 V, ½ F
and Pearl onions, *Birds Eye*	3.3 oz.	70	½ B, 1 V
and Pearl onions with cheese sauce, *Birds Eye*	5.0 oz.	160	1 B, ½ V, 1½ F
and Potatoes with cream sauce, *Birds Eye*	2.6 oz.	140	1 B, 1½ F
Shells, and corn, *Birds Eye*	3.3 oz.	130	1½ B, ½ F
Shells, and mushrooms, *Birds Eye*	3.3 oz.	130	1 B, ½ V, 1 F
with Sliced Mushrooms, *Birds Eye*	3.3 oz.	70	½ B, 1 V
Potatoes,			
Au gratin, *Stouffer's*	3¾ oz.	135	½ B, 1½ F, ½ Mk
Baked, stuffed, *Green Giant,*			
with Cheese-flavored topping	½ potato	180	1½ B, 1½ F
with Sour cream and chives	½ potato	240	1½ B, 3 F
Bites, *Tiny Taters*	3.2 oz	200	1½ B, 2 F
and Cheese pierogies, *Mrs. Paul's*	5 oz.	300	3½ B, ½ M, ½ F
Cottage fries, *Birds Eye*	2.8 oz.	120	1 B, 1 F
Crinkle cut, *Birds Eye*	3.0 oz.	110	1 B, 1 F
Farm-style Wedges, *Birds Eye*	3.0 oz.	10	1 B, 1 F
French fries,			
Birds Eye	3.0 oz.	110	1 B, 1 F
Tasti Fries	2.5 oz.	140	1 B, 1½ F
Hash browns, *Birds Eye*	4.0 oz.	70	1 B

Product Name	Serving Size	Calories	Exchanges
Puffs, *Tasti Puffs*	2.5 oz.	190	1½ B, 2 F
Scalloped, *Stouffer's*	4.0 oz.	125	1 B, 1½ F
Shoestrings, *Birds Eye*	3.3 oz.	140	1 B, 1½ F
Shredded hash browns, *Birds Eye*	3.0 oz.	60	1 B
Sliced, in butter sauce, *Green Giant*	½ cup	80	1 B, ½ F
Steak fries, *Birds Eye*	3.0 oz	110	1 B, 1 F
and Sweet peas in bacon cream sauce, *Green Giant*	½ cup	110	1 B, 1 F
Whole, peeled, *Birds Eye*	3.2 oz.	60	1 B
Ratatouille, *Stouffer's*	5.0 oz.	60	1½ V, ½ F
San Francisco Style with seasoned sauce, *Birds Eye*	3.3 oz.	50	½ B, ½ V
Spinach,			
Birds Eye,			
Chopped	3.3 oz.	20	1 V
Leaf	3.3 oz.	20	1 V
Harvest Fresh	½ cup	30	1 V
Almondine in pastry, *Pepperidge Farm*	1 piece	260	1 B, 1 V, 3½ F
in Butter sauce, *Green Giant*	½ cup	50	1 V, ½ F
Creamed,			
Birds Eye	3.0 oz.	60	1 V, ½ F
Stouffer's	4½ oz.	190	2 V, 3 F
in Cream sauce, *Green Giant*	½ cup	70	1 V, 1 F
Soufflé, *Stouffer's*	4.0 oz.	135	½ B, ½ M, 1 V, 1 F
and Water chestnuts, *Birds Eye*	3.3 oz.	30	1 V
Squash, *Birds Eye,*			
Cooked	4.0 oz.	45	½ B
Summer, sliced	3.3 oz.	18	½ V
Succotash, *Birds Eye*	3.3 oz.	90	1½ B
Turnip greens, *Birds Eye,*			
Chopped	3.3 oz.	20	1 V
with Diced turnips	3.3 oz.	20	1 V
Wax beans, cut, *Birds Eye*	3.0 oz.	25	1 V
Zucchini,			
Birds Eye	3.3 oz.	16	½ V
Provençal in pastry, *Pepperidge Farm*	1 piece	210	1 B, 1 V, 2½ F
Sticks, light batter, *Mrs. Paul's*	3.0 oz.	180	1 B, ½ V, 2 F

Product Name	Serving Size	Calories	Exchanges

■**Mixes—Potatoes**

Au gratin,

French's	½ cup prepared	150	1½ B, 1 F
General Mills	½ cup prepared	150	1½ B, 1 F
Libby's Potato Classics	¾ cup prepared	130	1½ B, ½ F
Creamed, *General Mills*	½ cup prepared	160	1½ B, 1½ F
Hash browns with onions, *General Mills*	½ cup prepared	150	1½ B, 1 F
Hickory-smoked cheese, *General Mills*	½ cup prepared	150	1½ B, 1 F
Julienne with mild cheese sauce, *General Mills*	½ cup prepared	130	1 B, 1½ F

Mashed,

American Beauty	½ cup prepared	120	1 B, 1 F
Country Store	⅓ cup flakes	70	1 B
French's,			
Big Tate	½ cup prepared	140	1 B, 1½ F
Idaho	½ cup prepared	120	1 B, 1 F
General Mills Potato Buds	½ cup prepared	130	1 B, 1½ F
Hungry Jack	½ cup prepared	140	1 B, 1½ F

Scalloped,

General Mills	½ cup prepared	140	1 B, 1½ F
Libby's Potato Classics	¾ cup prepared	130	1½ B, ½ F
with Cheese, *French's*	½ cup prepared	160	1½ B, 1½ F
Crispy top, *French's*	½ cup prepared	160	1½ B, 1½ F
Pancakes, *French's*	3 oz. prepared	130	1 B, 1 F

Sour cream and chive,

French's	½ cup prepared	170	1½ B, 1½ F
General Mills	½ cup prepared	140	1 B, 1½ F

4

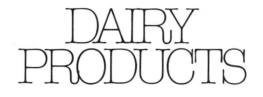

DAIRY PRODUCTS

☐ Butter and margarine

☐ Cheese

☐ Cream, nondairy creamers, and sour cream

☐ Milk

☐ Yogurt

Dairy products are made from milk and cream. Margarine and nondairy creamers, while not made from these items, are listed here for your convenience. You'll find that items in this chapter include meat and fat exchanges as well as milk exchanges.

The milk exchange list is based on *nonfat milk,* which includes only a trace of fat. Whole milk, "lowfat" milk, and products made from them do contain fat (1% to 3.5%), and you'll find them listed here with both fat and milk exchanges. Yogurts flavored with "extras" such as coffee, vanilla, and lemon contain small amounts of sugar as well; fruited yogurts high in sugar have been omitted.

Cream, sour cream, butter, and margarine are primarily fat (as much as 80%) and, thus, count as fat exchanges. Regular margarine has the same exchange value as butter, but is lower in saturated fat and has no cholesterol. Soft margarine is lower in saturated fat than stick margarine. If you are trying to lose weight, your exchange pattern will have few fat exchanges. You can stretch those exchanges by using whipped butter or margarine (about two-thirds the calories of regular margarine or butter, by volume) or imitation or diet margarine (about one-half the number of calories, by weight), and by substituting milk or half-and-half for cream.

Cheese, although made from milk, does not have milk's carbohydrate. It contains high-quality protein similar to that found in meat, as well as some additional fat. Thus, you'll find that most cheeses will correspond to meat and fat exchanges. Watch for the names "cheese food" and "cheese spread." These are *not* the same as natural cheese, and often contain preservatives and more salt.

Product Name	Serving Size	Calories	Exchanges
BUTTER AND MARGARINE			
Butter,			
Land O' Lakes,			
Lightly salted	1 tbsp.	100	2 F
Unsalted	1 tbsp.	100	2 F
Whipped, lightly salted	1 tbsp.	60	1½ F
Whipped, unsalted	1 tbsp.	60	1½ F
Margarine,			
Imitation, *Diet Mazola*	1 tbsp.	50	1 F
Stick,			
Chiffon	1 tbsp.	100	2 F
Cookman's Preservative-Free	1 tbsp.	100	2 F
Land O' Lakes	1 tbsp.	100	2 F
Land O' Lakes Country Morning Blend	1 tbsp.	100	2 F
Land O' Lakes Country Morning Blend, unsalted	1 tbsp.	100	2 F
Land O' Lakes **Corn Oil**	1 tbsp.	100	2 F
Mazola	1 tbsp.	105	2½ F
Mazola, **unsalted**	1 tbsp.	105	2½ F
Nucoa	1 tbsp.	105	2½ F
Weight Watchers, **reduced calorie**	1 tbsp.	60	1½ F
Soft,			
Chiffon	1 tbsp.	90	2 F
Chiffon, **unsalted**	1 tbsp.	90	2 F
Chiffon, **whipped**	1 tbsp.	70	1½ F
Land O' Lakes	1 tbsp.	100	2 F
Nucoa	1 tbsp.	90	2 F
Weight Watchers, **reduced calorie**	1 tbsp.	50	1 F
Weight Watchers, **reduced calorie, unsalted**	1 tbsp.	50	1 F

Product Name	Serving Size	Calories	Exchanges

CHEESE

■ Natural

American,

    Borden ... 1 oz. ... 110 ... 1 M, 1 F

    Land O' Lakes ... 1 oz. ... 110 ... 1 M, 1 F

American/Swiss, *Land O' Lakes* ... 1 oz. ... 100 ... 1 M, 1 F

Blue,

    Frigo ... 1 oz. ... 100 ... 1 M, 1 F

    Land O' Lakes ... 1 oz. ... 100 ... 1 M, 1 F

    Crumbled, *Treasure Cave* ... 1 oz. ... 100 ... 1 M, 1 F

Brick, *Land O' Lakes* ... 1 oz. ... 110 ... 1 M, 1 F

Cheddar,

    Featherweight **low sodium** ... 1 oz. ... 110 ... 1 M, 1 F

    Frigo ... 1 oz. ... 110 ... 1 M, 1 F

    Land O' Lakes ... 1 oz ... 110 ... 1 M, 1 F

    Pauly **low sodium** ... 1 oz. ... 110 ... 1 M, 1 F

Colby,

    Featherweight **low sodium** ... 1 oz. ... 110 ... 1 M, 1 F

    Land O' Lakes ... 1 oz. ... 110 ... 1 M, 1 F

    Pauly **low sodium** ... 1 oz. ... 110 ... 1 M, 1 F

Cottage cheese,

    Borden **4% milkfat** ... ½ cup ... 120 ... 2 M

    Borden Lite-line **lowfat** ... ½ cup ... 90 ... 1½ M

    Land O' Lakes ... 4 oz. ... 120 ... 2 M

    Land O' Lakes **2%** ... 4 oz. ... 113 ... 2 M

    Weight Watchers **lowfat** ... ⅓ cup ... 60 ... 1 M

Cream cheese, imitation,
  Weight Watchers ... ⅓ cup ... 60 ... 1 M

Edam, *Land O' Lakes* ... 1 oz. ... 100 ... 1 M, 1 F

Feta, *Frigo* ... 1 oz. ... 100 ... 1 M, 1 F

Gouda, *Land O' Lakes* ... 1 oz. ... 100 ... 1 M, 1 F

Monterey Jack, *Land O' Lakes* ... 1 oz. ... 110 ... 1 M, 1 F

Mozzarella,

  Part skim,

    Frigo ... 1 oz. ... 80 ... 1 M, ½ F

    Land O' Lakes ... 1 oz. ... 80 ... 1 M, ½ F

  Whole milk, *Frigo* ... 1 oz. ... 90 ... 1 M, ½ F

Muenster, *Land O' Lakes* ... 1 oz. ... 100 ... 1 M, 1 F

Parmesan,

  Frigo,

    Grated ... 1 oz. ... 130 ... 1½ M, 1 F

Product Name	Serving Size	Calories	Exchanges
Loaf	1 oz.	110	1½ M, ½ F
and Romano, *Frigo,* grated	1 oz.	130	1½ M, 1 F
Part skim milk, *Weight Watchers*	1 oz.	80	1 M, ½ F
Provolone,			
Frigo	1 oz	90	1 M, ½ F
Land O' Lakes	1 oz.	100	1 M, 1 F
Ricotta,			
Part skim,			
Frigo	½ cup	170	2 M, 1 F
Sorrento	4 oz.	190	2 M, 1½ F
Whole milk,			
Frigo	½ cup	215	2 M, 2 F
Sorrento	4 oz.	213	2 M, 2 F
Romano,			
Frigo,			
Grated	1 oz.	130	1½ M, 1 F
Loaf	1 oz.	110	1 M, 1 F
Land O' Lakes, grated	1 oz.	130	1½ M, 1 F
Swiss,			
Frigo	1 oz.	110	1 M, 1 F
Land O' Lakes	1 oz.	110	1 M, 1 F

■ Cheese Foods and Spreads

Product Name	Serving Size	Calories	Exchanges
Cheese food,			
All flavors, *Borden Lite-line*	1 oz.	50	1 M
American, *Borden*	1 oz.	90	1 M, 1 F
Blue, *Wispride*	1 oz.	100	1 M, 1 F
Caraway, *Land O' Lakes*	1 oz.	90	1 M, ½ F
Cheddar flavor, *Wispride*	1 oz.	90	1 M, ½ F
Cheese 'N Salami, *Land O' Lakes*	1 oz.	100	1 M, 1 F
Hot pepper, *Land O'Lakes*	1 oz.	90	1 M, ½ F
Land O' Lakes,			
LaChedda	1 oz.	90	1 M, ½ F
Ole Smoky	1 oz.	90	1 M, ½ F
Low cholesterol substitute, *Borden Lite-line*	1 oz.	90	1 M, ½ F
Pimiento, *Land O' Lakes*	1 oz.	110	1 M, 1 F
Pizza-Pepperoni, *Land O' Lakes*	1 oz.	90	1 M, ½ F
Port wine, *Wispride*	1 oz.	100	1 M, 1 F
Royal American, *Land O' Lakes*	1 oz.	90	1 M, ½ F
Sharp cheddar, *Land O' Lakes*	1 oz.	90	1 M, ½ F

Product Name	Serving Size	Calories	Exchanges
Smoked, *Wispride*	1 oz.	90	1 M, ½ F
Swiss, *Borden*	1 oz.	100	1 M, 1 F
Tangy onion, *Land O' Lakes*	1 oz.	90	1 M, ½ F
Weight Watchers	1 oz.	50	1 M
Cheese spread,			
Snack Mate,			
American	4 tsp.	60	1 M
Cheddar	4 tsp.	60	1 M
Cheddar, sharp	4 tsp.	60	1 M
Cheese 'N' Bacon	4 tsp.	60	1 M
Chive 'N' Green Onion	4 tsp.	60	1 M
Land O' Lakes Golden Velvet	1 oz.	80	1 M, ½ F
Price's **Pimiento spread**	1 oz.	80	½ M, 1 F
Swiss Knight **fondue**	1 oz.	60	½ M, ½ F

CREAM, NONDAIRY CREAMERS, AND SOUR CREAM

Product Name	Serving Size	Calories	Exchanges
Cream, whipping, *Land O' Lakes*	1 tbsp.	45	1 F
Half and half, *Land O' Lakes*	1 tbsp.	20	½ F
Nondairy creamer,			
Coffee-Mate	1 tsp.	10	free in moderation
Coffee Rich	1 tsp.	7	free in moderation
Poly Rich	1 tsp	7	free in moderation
Sour cream,			
Land O' Lakes	1 tbsp.	25	½ F
Imitation, *Pet*	1 tbsp.	25	½ F

MILK

Product Name	Serving Size	Calories	Exchanges
Buttermilk,			
Borden	1 cup	90	1 Mk
Land O' Lakes	1 cup	100	½ F, 1 Mk
Evaporated milk,			
Carnation	½ cup	170	2 F, 1 Mk
Pet	½ cup	170	2 F, 1 Mk
Filled, *Dairymate*	½ cup	150	1½ F, 1 Mk
Lowfat, *Carnation*	½ cup	110	½ F, 1 Mk
Skimmed,			
Carnation	½ cup	100	1 Mk
Pet	½ cup	100	1 Mk

Product Name	Serving Size	Calories	Exchanges
Lowfat milk,			
Land O' Lakes, 1%	1 cup	100	½ F, 1 Mk
Land O' Lakes, 2%	1 cup	120	1 F, 1 Mk
Nonfat milk, instant,			
Carnation	1 cup prepared	80	1 Mk
Land O' Lakes Flash	1 cup prepared	80	1 Mk
Borden Skim-line, protein fortified	1 cup prepared	100	½ M, 1 Mk
Skim milk,			
Land O' Lakes	1 cup	90	1 Mk
Weight Watchers	1 cup	90	1 Mk
Whole milk, *Land O' Lakes*	1 cup	150	1½ F, 1 Mk

YOGURT

Flavored, *Dannon* (coffee, vanilla, lemon)	8 oz.	200	1½ B, ½ F, 1 Mk
Fruited, *Weight Watchers,* **nonfat** (blueberry, raspberry, strawberry)	1 cup	150	1½ Fr, 1 Mk
Plain,			
Borden Lite-line **lowfat**	8 oz.	180	½ F, 2 Mk
Dannon	8 oz.	150	½ F, 1½ Mk
Yoplait	6 oz.	130	1 F, 1 Mk
Weight Watchers **nonfat**	1 cup	90	1 Mk

5

BAKED GOODS, CEREALS, GRAIN PRODUCTS

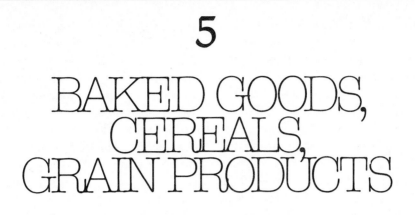

☐ Biscuits, muffins, and rolls
☐ Bread
☐ Breadsticks
☐ Cake
☐ Cereal
☐ Chips, puffs, and snacks
☐ Cookies and bars
☐ Crackers
☐ Croutons, crumbs, and crusts
☐ Pancakes, waffles, and French toast
☐ Pasta
☐ Rice
☐ Stuffing

Foods in this chapter are made from grains (barley, corn, oats, rice, rye, and wheat). Grain foods are composed of a small amount of protein and the same kind of complex carbohydrate found in peas, beans, lentils, potatoes, and other starchy vegetables (see Chapter 3). Since many physicians and dietitians recommend that these complex-carbohydrate foods make up 50% to 60% of the calories in your daily meal plan, your ADA diet has been calculated with this in mind.

All of these foods contain bread exchanges; certain highly processed foods also contain fat exchanges. Exchanges for some breads and rolls may not correspond to those given in the ADA or other exchange lists. Standard exchange lists give *average* values; the exchanges listed here are more exact because they're based on actual nutrients. The exchange for a given bread may be closer to one-and-a-half or one-half than to one, while rolls or muffins may contain enough fat to equal a fat exchange. Many cereals contain added sugar. We've listed here only those that are not highly sweetened. Granola-type cereals contain fat from oils and nuts, and have fat exchanges that must be counted. Because of their concentrated calories, you'll find that the serving size for granola cereals is usually quite small.

When selecting foods, you'll want to consider not only the exchanges but also the amount of fiber and salt. Many chips, snacks, crackers, and seasoned rices and pastas contain substantial amounts of salt. Whole-grain breads, muffins, and rolls; bran and high-fiber cereals; and brown rice all contain substantial amounts of dietary fiber, which improves blood cholesterol levels and bowel function. Highly processed foods, such as those made from white flour, lack this ingredient.

Researchers are just beginning to study the effects of complex carbohydrates on blood sugar levels. Until recently, they assumed that *all* complex carbohydrate foods (that is, all foods in the bread exchange group) had a similar effect—a relatively minor increase in blood sugar levels when compared to the effects of simple sugars. Recent work, however, has suggested that items equal in bread exchanges (containing equal amounts of calories and carbohydrate) may *not* affect

blood sugar levels in the same way.[*] Bread, pasta, and rice, for instance, have different effects, some of which overlap those of simple sugars. However, until further research is conducted, these foods will still be grouped together in the bread exchange list. The American Diabetes Association is considering subdividing the bread exchange list into categories that reflect the different effects of foods on blood sugar levels.

Similar research has also suggested that a modest amount of sucrose (table sugar) eaten as part of a balanced meal may not lead to higher blood sugar levels than does consumption of some complex-carbohydrate foods.[**] In light of this (and particularly if you are monitoring your blood sugar level at home and keeping it within normal limits) your physician may let you work limited amounts of sugar-sweetened foods into your meal plan. However, unless you're a well-controlled insulin-dependent diabetic using these foods during vigorous exercise, you should not eat these foods between meals, nor substitute them indiscriminately for complex-carbohydrate foods containing fewer calories, more fiber, and other important nutrients.

With the expectation that restrictions on sugar-sweetened foods may be relaxed somewhat, some cookies and cakes have been included here, marked with an asterisk for your convenience and calculated as bread exchanges. We've included relatively few of these items, and the presence of a particular item does not imply its endorsement. Very sweet foods such as iced and frosted cakes, pastries, and pies are omitted, because, regardless of their effect on blood sugar, these items are very high in calories and low in nutrients

[*]Jenkins, D., Wolever, T., Taylor, R., *et al. Am. J. Clin. Nutr.* 34:362,1981.
[**]Bantle, J.P., *et al. New Engl. J. Med.*309:7,1983.

and fiber. For lists of cookies, cakes, and other items sweetened with aspartame (NutraSweet), fructose, saccharin, and sorbitol, see Chapter 8.

Product Name	Serving Size	Calories	Exchanges

BISCUITS, MUFFINS, AND ROLLS

Biscuits,

Product Name	Serving Size	Calories	Exchanges
Ballard Oven-ready	2 biscuits	100	1½ B
Merico Butter-Me-Not	1 biscuit	90	½ B, 1 F
Wonder	1 biscuit	100	1 B, ½ F
Baking powder,			
1869 Brand	2 biscuits	190	2 B, 1 F
Tenderflake	2 biscuits	110	1 B, 1 F
Butter,			
1869 Brand	2 biscuits	190	2 B, 1 F
Hungry Jack Flaky	2 biscuits	190	1½ B, 2 F
Pillsbury	2 biscuits	100	1½ B
Pillsbury Big Country	2 biscuits	190	2 B, 1 F
Buttermilk,			
Ballard Oven-ready	2 biscuits	100	1½ B
1869 Brand	2 biscuits	190	2 B, 1 F
Hungry Jack Extra Rich	2 biscuits	130	1 B, 1½ F
Hungry Jack Flaky	2 biscuits	170	1½ B, 1½ F
Hungry Jack Fluffy	2 biscuits	180	1½ B, 2 F
Pillsbury	2 biscuits	100	1½ B
Pillsbury Big Country	2 biscuits	200	2 B, 1½ F
Pillsbury Big Premium	2 biscuits	270	2 B, 3 F
Pillsbury Country Style	2 biscuits	100	1½ B
Pillsbury Extra Lights	2 biscuits	110	1 B, 1 F
Pillsbury Heat 'n Eat	2 biscuits	170	2 B, 1 F
Tenderflake	2 biscuits	110	1 B, 1 F
Weight Watchers Ready-to-bake	2 biscuits	80	1 B
Flaky, *Hungry Jack*	2 biscuits	180	1½ B, 2 F
Mix, *Bisquick*	½ cup	240	2½ B, 1½ F
Wheat, *Weight Watchers Ready-to-bake*	2 biscuits	80	1 B
Dinner rolls,			
Home Pride	1 roll	85	1 B, ½ F
Pepperidge Farm	1 roll	60	1 B
Butter Crescent, *Pepperidge Farm Heat & Serve*	1 roll	110	1 B, 1 F

Product Name	Serving Size	Calories	Exchanges
Butterflake, *Pillsbury*	1 roll	110	1 B, 1 F
with Buttermilk, *Wonder Brown 'n Serve*	1 roll	85	1 B, ½ F
Club, *Pepperidge Farm Brown and Serve*	1 roll	100	1½ B
Country White, *Pillsbury*	1 roll	90	1 B, ½ F
Crescent, *Pillsbury*	2 rolls	200	1½ B, 2 F
Finger, with poppy seeds, *Pepperidge Farm*	1 roll	60	½ B, ½ F
French,			
Pepperidge Farm	1 roll	110	1½ B
Pepperidge Farm Brown and Serve (**2 roll pkg.**)	½ roll	190	2½ B, ½ F
Pepperidge Farm Brown and Serve (**3 roll pkg.**)	½ roll	130	2 B
Wonder Brown 'n Serve	1 roll	75	1 B
Sour, *Pepperidge Farm*	1 roll	100	1½ B
Sourdough, *Francisco*	1 roll	90	1½ B
Gem Style, *Wonder Brown 'n Serve*	1 roll	85	1 B, ½ F
Golden Twist, *Pepperidge Farm Brown and Serve*	1 roll	120	1 B, 1 F
Half and Half, *Wonder Brown 'n Serve*	1 roll	80	1 B
Hearth, *Pepperidge Farm Brown and Serve*	1 roll	80	1 B
Home Bake, *Wonder Brown 'n Serve*	1 roll	85	1 B, ½ F
Home Style, dough, *Rich's*	2 rolls	150	2 B, ½ F
Mix, *Pillsbury*	2 rolls, prepared	200	2½ B, ½ F
Parker House,			
Pepperidge Farm	1 roll	60	½ B, ½ F
Pillsbury	2 rolls	150	1½ B, 1 F
Party Rounds, *Arnold*	2 rolls	110	1½ B
Soft Family, *Pepperidge Farm*	1 roll	110	1½ B
English muffins,			
Arnold Extra Crisp	1 muffin	150	2 B, ½ F
Bran'nola	1 muffin	160	2½ B
Pepperidge Farm	1 muffin	140	2 B
Thomas'	1 muffin	130	2 B
Wonder	1 muffin	130	2 B
Cinnamon apple, *Pepperidge Farm*	1 muffin	140	2 B

Product Name	Serving Size	Calories	Exchanges
Cinnamon raisin,			
Pepperidge Farm	1 muffin	150	2 B, ½ F
Honey wheat, *Thomas'*	1 muffin	130	2 B
Raisin,			
Arnold	1 muffin	170	2½ B
Wonder Raisin Rounds	1 muffin	150	2 B, ½ F
Sourdough,			
Pepperidge Farm	1 muffin	140	2 B
Thomas'	1 muffin	130	2 B
Wonder	1 muffin	130	2 B
Wheat, *Pepperidge Farm*	1 muffin	130	2 B
Frankfurter rolls, *Pepperidge Farm*	1 roll	110	1½ B
Hamburger buns,			
Arnold	1 roll	110	1½ B
Pepperidge Farm	1 roll	130	2 B
Wonder	1 roll	120	2 B
Hot dog buns, *Arnold*	1 roll	110	1½ B
Muffins,			
Blueberry,			
Pepperidge Farm	1 muffin	180	2 B, 1 F
Thomas' Toast-r-Cakes	1 muffin	112	1 B, 1 F
Mix, *General Mills*	1 muffin, prepared	120	1 B, 1 F
Bran,			
Thomas' Toast-r-Cakes	1 muffin	115	1 B, 1 F
with Raisin, *Pepperidge Farm*	1 muffin	180	2 B, 1 F
Corn,			
Pepperidge Farm	1 muffin	180	2 B, 1 F
Thomas' Toast-r-Cakes	1 muffin	110	1 B, 1 F
Mix, *Dromedary*	1 muffin, prepared	130	1½ B, 1 F
Mix, *Flako*	1 muffin, prepared	140	1½ B, 1 F
Mix, *General Mills*	1 muffin, prepared	160	1½ B, 1 F
Orange-cranberry, *Pepperidge Farm*	1 muffin	190	2 B, 1 F
Popover mix, *Flako*	1 popover	170	2 B, 1 F
Sandwich buns,			
Dutch Egg, *Arnold*	1 roll	130	2 B
French style, *Francisco*	1 roll	160	2½ B
Hoagie roll, *Wonder*	1 roll	460	5½ B, 1½ F
Kaiser roll, *Wonder*	1 roll	460	5½ B, 1½ F
Onion with poppy seeds, *Pepperidge Farm*	1 roll	150	2 B, ½ F

Product Name	Serving Size	Calories	Exchanges
with Poppy seeds, *Pepperidge Farm*	1 roll	130	1½ B, ½ F
with Sesame seeds, *Pepperidge Farm*	1 roll	130	1½ B, ½ F
Soft, plain, with poppy seeds, or sesame seeds, *Arnold*	1 roll	110	1½ B

BREAD

Apple with cinnamon, *Pepperidge Farm*	1 slice	70	1 B
Bran,			
with Diced raisins, *Pepperidge Farm*	1 slice	65	1 B
Honey, *Pepperidge Farm*	1 slice	95	1 B, ½ F
Brown,			
Plain, canned,			
B & M	½-inch slice	80	1 B
Friend's	½-inch slice	80	1 B
with Raisins, canned,			
B & M	½-inch slice	80	1 B
Friend's	½-inch slice	80	1 B
Cinnamon, *Pepperidge Farm*	1 slice	80	1 B
Corn,			
Mix,			
Aunt Jemima	⅙ loaf, prepared	220	2 B, 1½ F
Ballard	⅛ pkg., prepared	140	1½ B, ½ F
Dromedary	2" × 2" square, prepared	130	1½ B, 1 F
and Molasses, *Pepperidge Farm*	1 slice	75	1 B
Date walnut, *Pepperidge Farm*	1 slice	75	1 B
French,			
Francisco, unsliced	1 oz.	80	1 B
Pepperidge Farm,			
Brown and Serve	1 oz.	90	1½ B
Fully Baked	1 oz.	75	1 B
Wonder	1 slice	75	1 B
Vienna, *Francisco*, unsliced	1 oz.	80	1 B
Italian, *Pepperidge Farm* Brown and Serve	1 oz.	75	1 B
Mixed grain,			
Hillbilly	1 slice	70	1 B
Hollywood,			
Dark	1 slice	70	1 B

Product Name	Serving Size	Calories	Exchanges
Light	1 slice	70	1 B
Home Pride Seven-Grain	1 slice	70	1 B
Roman Meal	1 slice	70	1 B
Oat, *Bran'nola*	1 slice	110	1½ B
Oatmeal, *Pepperidge Farm*	1 slice	70	1 B
Pocket,			
Sahara	1 mini pocket	80	1 B
Wheat, *Sahara*	1 mini pocket	75	1 B
Protein, *Thomas'*	1 slice	47	½ B
Pumpernickel,			
Arnold	1 slice	75	1 B
Levy	1 slice	85	1 B
Pepperidge Farm,			
Family	1 slice	85	1 B
Party Slices	4 slices	70	1 B
Quickbread, mix, *Pillsbury,* *			
Applesauce spice	¹⁄₁₂ loaf, prepared	150	1 B, 1 F, 1 Fr
Apricot nut	¹⁄₁₂ loaf, prepared	160	1 B, 1 F, 1 Fr
Banana	¹⁄₁₂ loaf, prepared	150	1 B, 1 F, 1 Fr
Blueberry nut	¹⁄₁₂ loaf, prepared	150	1 B, 1 F, 1 Fr
Carrot nut	¹⁄₁₂ loaf, prepared	150	1½ B, 1 F
Cherry nut	¹⁄₁₂ loaf, prepared	170	1½ B, 1 F, ½ Fr
Cranberry	¹⁄₁₂ loaf, prepared	160	1 B, 1 F, 1 Fr
Date nut	¹⁄₁₂ loaf, prepared	160	1 B, 1 F, 1 Fr
Raisin,			
with Cinnamon, *Pepperidge Farm*	1 slice	75	1 B
Tea, *Arnold*	1 slice	70	1 B
Rye,			
Continental,			
Hearty	1 slice	70	1 B
Mild	1 slice	70	1 B
Pepperidge Farm,			
Family	1 slice	85	1 B
Party Slices	4 slices	70	1 B
Seedless	1 slice	85	1 B
Very Thin Sliced	1 slice	45	½ B
Weight Watchers Soft Light	1 slice	40	½ B
Dill, *Arnold*	1 slice	75	1 B

*Contains sugar.

Product Name	Serving Size	Calories	Exchanges

Jewish,

Arnold, seeded or unseeded	1 slice	75	1 B
Levy, seeded or unseeded	1 slice	80	1 B
Pepperidge Farm	1 slice	90	1½ B
Melba Thin, *Arnold*	1 slice	50	½ B
Sourdough, *DiCarlo*	1 slice	70	1 B

Taco shell,

Old El Paso	1 shell	50	½ B, ½ F
Ortega	1 shell	50	½ B, ½ F

Tortilla,

Corn, *El Charrito*	2 tortillas	45	½ B
Flour, *El Charrito*	2 tortillas	180	2 B, 1 F

Vienna, thick sliced,

Pepperidge Farm	1 slice	75	1 B

Wheat,

Arnold,

Brick Oven, 16 oz.pkg.	1 slice	60	1 B
Brick Oven, 32 oz. pkg.	1 slice	80	1 B
Measure Up	1 slice	40	½ B
Bran'nola	1 slice	90	1½ B
Hearty	1 slice	105	1½ B
Fresh Horizons	1 slice	50	½ B
Fresh & Natural	1 slice	70	1 B

Pepperidge Farm,

1½ lb.	1 slice	95	1½ B
Sandwich	1 slice	55	1 B
Wonder, **Family**	1 slice	75	1 B
Butter top, *Home Pride*	1 slice	75	1 B

Cracked wheat,

Pepperidge Farm	1 slice	75	1 B
Weight Watchers	1 slice	40	½ B
Wonder	1 slice	75	1 B

Honey wheat,

Home Pride	1 slice	70	1 B
Dough, *Rich's*	1 slice, baked	60	1 B

Honey wheatberry,

Arnold	1 slice	90	1½ B
Home Pride	1 slice	70	1 B
Pepperidge Farm	1 slice	55	1 B

Sprouted wheat,

Arnold	1 slice	65	1 B

Product Name	Serving Size	Calories	Exchanges
Pepperidge Farm	1 slice	70	1 B
Stone ground, *Arnold*	1 slice	55	1 B
Wheatberry, *Home Pride*	1 slice	70	1 B
Wheat germ, *Pepperidge Farm*	1 slice	70	1 B
Whole wheat, 100%,			
Home Pride	1 slice	70	1 B
Pepperidge Farm	1 slice	70	1 B
Pepperidge Farm Very Thin Sliced	1 slice	70	1 B
White,			
Arnold,			
Brick Oven, 16 oz. pkg.	1 slice	65	1 B
Brick Oven, 32 oz. pkg.	1 slice	85	1 B
Country	1 slice	95	1½ B
Hearthstone	1 slice	85	1 B
Measure Up	1 slice	40	½ B
Bran'nola Old Style	1 slice	105	1½ B
Fresh Horizons	1 slice	50	½ B
Pepperidge Farm,			
Large Family Thin Sliced	1 slice	75	1 B
Sandwich	1 slice	65	1 B
Thin Sliced	1 slice	75	1 B
Toasting White	1 slice	85	1 B
Very Thin	1 slice	45	½ B
Weight Watchers Old Fashioned	1 slice	40	½ B
Wonder	1 slice	70	1 B
Butter top, *Home Pride*	1 slice	75	1 B
with Buttermilk, *Wonder*	1 slice	75	1 B
with Cracked wheat, *Pepperidge Farm*	1 slice	95	1½ B
Dough,			
Pillsbury Pipin' Hot Loaf	1-inch slice, baked	80	1 B
Rich's	2 slices, baked	120	2 B

BREADSTICKS

Product Name	Serving Size	Calories	Exchanges
Cheese, *Lance*	1 oz.	110	1½ B
Garlic, *Lance*	1 oz.	110	1½ B
Onion,			
Lance	1 oz.	110	1½ B
Stella D'Oro	1 piece	40	½ B
Plain, *Stella D'Oro*	1 piece	43	½ B

Product Name	Serving Size	Calories	Exchanges
Salted, *Lance*	1 oz.	110	1½ B
Sesame, *Stella D'Oro*	1 piece	52	½ B, ½ F
White, soft, dough, *Pillsbury Pipin' Hot*	1 stick	100	1 B, ½ F
Whole wheat, *Stella D'Oro*	1 piece	40	½ B

CAKE

Angel food, mix,			
*Betty Crocker One-Step**	½12 cake, prepared	140	2 B
*Betty Crocker Traditional**	½12 cake, prepared	130	2 B
*Pillsbury**	½24 cake, prepared	70	1 B
Chocolate, *Betty Crocker**	½12 cake, prepared	140	2 B
Confetti, *Betty Crocker**	½12 cake, prepared	150	2 B
Lemon Custard, *Betty Crocker**	½12 cake, prepared	140	2 B
Strawberry, *Betty Crocker**	½12 cake, prepared	150	2 B
Applesauce raisin, mix, *Snackin' Cake**	⅑ cake, prepared	180	2 B, 1 F
Banana walnut, mix, *Snackin' Cake**	⅑ cake, prepared	190	2 B, 1 F
Carrot nut, mix, *Snackin' Cake**	⅑ cake, prepared	180	2 B, 1 F
Chocolate almond, mix, *Snackin' Cake**	⅑ cake, prepared	190	2 B, 1 F
Chocolate chip, mix, *Snackin' Cake**	⅑ cake, prepared	190	2 B, 1 F
Chocolate fudge chip, mix, *Snackin' Cake**	⅑ cake, prepared	190	2 B, 1 F
Coconut pecan, mix, *Snackin' Cake**	⅑ cake, prepared	190	2 B, 1 F
Date nut, mix, *Snackin' Cake**	⅑ cake, prepared	190	2 B, 1 F
German chocolate coconut pecan, mix, *Snackin' Cake**	⅑ cake, prepared	190	2 B, 1 F
Gingerbread, mix, *Dromedary**	2″ × 2″ square, prepared	100	1 B, ½ F
Lemon chiffon, *Betty Crocker**	½12 cake, prepared	190	2 B, 1 F
Pound,			
Butter, *Pepperidge Farm**	1 oz.	130	1 B, 1½ F
Mix,			
*Betty Crocker**	½12 cake, prepared	200	1½ B, 2 F
*Dromedary**	¾-inch slice, prepared	210	2 B, 2 F
Spice raisin, mix, *Snackin' Cake**	⅑ cake, prepared	180	2 B, 1 F

*Contains sugar.

Product Name	Serving Size	Calories	Exchanges

CEREAL

■ Cooked

Barley, pearled,			
Quaker Scotch Brand	1 cup, prepared	170	2½ B
Cream of Wheat,	2½ tbsp., dry	100	1½ B
Instant	2½ tbsp., dry	100	1½ B
Mix 'n Eat, **regular**	1 pkg.	100	1½ B
Quick	2½ tbsp., dry	100	1½ B
Farina, *Pillsbury*	⅔ cup, prepared	80	1 B
Grits,			
Instant, *Quaker,*	1 pkg.	80	1 B
with **Artificial cheese flavor**	1 pkg.	100	1½ B
with **Imitation bacon bits**	1 pkg.	100	1½ B
with **Imitation ham bits**	1 pkg.	100	1½ B
White hominy,			
Aunt Jemima	3 tbsp., dry	100	1½ B
Quaker	3 tbsp., dry	100	1½ B
Hominy,			
Golden, *Van Camp*	8 oz., prepared	120	2 B
White, *Van Camp*	8 oz., prepared	125	2 B
Oatmeal,			
Quaker Oats	⅔ cup, prepared	110	1½ B
Ralston Quick Oats	⅓ cup, dry	110	1½ B
Instant, *Quaker,*	1 pkg.	110	1½ B
with **Apples and cinnamon***	1 pkg.	140	2 B
with **Bran and raisins***	1 pkg.	150	2 B
with **Honey and graham***	1 pkg.	140	2 B
with **Raisins and spice***	1 pkg.	160	2½ B
Whole wheat,			
Quaker Pettijohns	⅔ cup, prepared	100	1½ B
Ralston, **instant or regular**	¼ cup, dry	100	1½ B

■ Dry, Ready-to-Eat

Bran or fiber,			
Bran Chex	⅔ cup	90	1½ B
Fruit & Fibre,			
Apples and Cinnamon	1 oz.	90	1½ B
Dates, Raisins, Walnuts	1 oz.	90	1½ B

*Contains sugar.

Product Name	Serving Size	Calories	Exchanges
General Foods,			
40% Bran Flakes	1 oz.	90	1½ B
Raisin Bran	1 oz.	90	1½ B
Kellogg's,			
All-Bran®	1 oz. (about ⅓ cup)	70	1 B
Bran Buds®	1 oz. (about ⅓ cup)	70	1 B
40% Bran Flakes	1 oz. (about ⅔ cup)	90	1½ B
Most®	1 oz. (about ½ cup)	100	1½ B
Raisin Bran	1.3 oz. (about ¾ cup)	110	1½ B
Nabisco **100% Bran**	6 tbsp.	53	1 B
Ralston,			
40% Bran Flakes	¾ cup	100	1½ B
Raisin Bran	¾ cup	120	2 B
Corn,			
Corn Chex	1 cup	110	1½ B
Corn Total	1 cup	110	1½ B
Country **Corn Flakes**	1 cup	110	1½ B
Featherweight **Corn Flakes**	1 oz.	110	1½ B
Kellogg's Corn Flakes®	1 oz.	110	1½ B
Kix	1½ cups	110	1½ B
Nutri-Grain™ **Corn**	1 oz. (about ½ cup)	110	1½ B
Post Toasties	1 oz.	110	1½ B
Ralston **Corn Flakes**	1 cup	110	1½ B
Granola,			
C.W. Post,			
Hearty	1 oz.	130	1½ B, ½ F
with Raisins	1 oz.	120	1½ B, ½ F
Heartland,			
Coconut	¼ cup	130	1 B, 1½ F
Plain	¼ cup	130	1 B, 1½ F
Raisin	¼ cup	130	1 B, 1½ F
Quaker **100% Natural**	¼ cup	140	1½ B, 1 F
with Apples and cinnamon	¼ cup	140	1½ B, 1 F
with Raisins and dates	¼ cup	130	1½ B, 1 F
Mixed-grain,			
Grape-Nuts	1 oz.	100	1½ B
Flakes	1 oz.	100	1½ B
Raisin	1 oz.	100	1½ B
Kellogg's,			
Product 19®	1 oz. (about ¾ cup)	110	1½ B

Product Name	Serving Size	Calories	Exchanges
Raisins, Rice, and Rye™	1.3 oz. (about ¾ cup)	140	2 B
Special K®	1 oz. (about 1 cup)	110	1½ B
Team Flakes	⅔ cup	69	1 B
Oat,			
Cheerios	1¼ cups	110	1½ B
General Foods Fortified Oat Flakes	1 oz.	100	1½ B
Tasteeos	1¼ cup	110	1½ B
Rice,			
Featherweight **Milled Rice**	1 oz.	110	1½ B
Kellogg's Rice Krispies®	1 oz. (about 1 cup)	110	1½ B
Quaker Puffed Rice	1 cup	50	½ B
Ralston Crispy Rice	1 cup	110	1½ B
Rice Chex	1⅛ cup	110	1½ B
Wheat,			
Featherweight **Wheat Flakes**	1 oz.	100	1½ B
Nabisco,			
Shredded Wheat	1 biscuit	90	1½ B
Spoon Size Shredded Wheat	½ cup	80	1 B
Nutri-Grain™ **Wheat**	1 oz. (about ⅔ cup)	110	1½ B
and Raisins	1.4 oz. (about ⅔ cup)	140	2 B
Quaker,			
Puffed Wheat	1 cup	50	½ B
Shredded Wheat	2 biscuits	140	2 B
Total	1 cup	110	1½ B
Wheat Chex	⅔ cup	110	1½ B
Wheat and Raisin Chex	¾ cup	130	2 B
Wheaties	1 cup	110	1½ B
Wheat germ, *Kretschmer*	¼ cup	110	1 B, 1 F

CHIPS, PUFFS, AND SNACKS

Cheese,			
Balls, baked, *Guy's*	1 oz.	160	1 B, 2 F
Cheddar chips, *Flavor Tree*	1 oz.	160	1 B, 2 F
Curls,			
Borden Lite-line	1 oz.	130	1½ B, 1 F
Featherweight **reduced sodium** . .	1 oz.	150	1 B, 2 F
Flavored baked corn puffs, *Cheez Doodles*	1 oz.	160	1 B, 2 F
Flavored fried corn puffs, *Cheez Doodles*	1 oz.	160	1 B, 2 F

Product Name	Serving Size	Calories	Exchanges
Flavored snack,			
Cheese 'N Crunch	1 oz.	161	1 B, 2 F
Twists,			
Bachman Baked Jax	1 oz.	150	1 B, 2 F
Bachman Crunchy Jax	1 oz.	160	1 B, 2 F
Lance	1 pkg. (1 oz.)	166	1 B, 2 F
Corn,			
Chips,			
Bachman	1 oz.	150	1 B, 2 F
Bachman Bar-B-Que	1 oz.	150	1 B, 2 F
Featherweight **low sodium**	1 oz.	170	1 B, 2 F
Lance	1 pkg. (1¾ oz.)	260	1½ B, 3½ F
Crunchies, *Wise*	1 oz.	160	1 B, 2 F
Curls, *Flings*	16 pieces	162	1 B, 2 F
and Sesame chips, *Nabisco*	16 pieces	160	1 B, 2 F
Snacks, *Bugles*	1 oz.	150	1 B, 1½ F
Mixed snacks, *Doo Dads*	57 pieces	140	1 B, 1½ F
Nut and snack mix, *Flavor Tree*	1 oz.	160	½ B, ½ M, 2 F
Popcorn,			
Bachman	1 oz.	160	1 B, 2 F
Hungry Jack,			
Butter flavor microwave	4 cups popped	260	2 B, 3 F
Microwave	4 cups popped	280	2 B, 3 F
Lance	1 pkg. (1 oz.)	141	1 B, 1½ F
Butter flavor, *Wise*	½ oz.	70	½ B, 1 F
Cheese,			
Bachman	1 oz.	180	1 B, 2½ F
Wise Cheez	½ oz.	90	½ B, 1 F
Popcorn flavored snack,			
Corn Diggers	36 pieces	151	1 B, 2 F
Pork skins, *Lance*	1 pkg. (½ oz.)	78	1 M, ½ F
Potato chips,			
Bachman	1 oz.	160	1 B, 2 F
Lance	1 pkg. (1¼ oz.)	215	1 B, 3 F
Wise	1 oz.	160	1 B, 2 F
Barbecue,			
Bachman BBQ	1 oz.	150	1 B, 2 F
Morton's Ridgies	1 oz.	150	1 B, 2 F
Ketchup and french fry, *Buckeye*	1 oz.	160	1 B, 2 F
Sour cream and onion, *Bachman*	1 oz.	150	1 B, 2 F
Unsalted,			
Bachman	1 oz.	160	1 B, 2 F

Product Name	Serving Size	Calories	Exchanges
Featherweight	1 oz.	160	1 B, 2 F
Vinegar, *Bachman*	1 oz.	150	1 B, 2 F
Potato sticks, O&C	1½ oz.	231	1½ B, 3 F
Pretzels,			
Bachman,	1 oz.	110	1½ B
Butter Twist	1 oz.	110	1½ B
Low salt	1 oz.	110	1½ B
Estee, **unsalted**	15 pretzels	75	1 B
Featherweight, **unsalted**	3 pretzels	20	½ B
Mr. Salty	4 pretzels	80	1 B
Pretz-L Nuggets	1 oz.	110	1½ B
Rokeach	1 oz.	110	1½ B
Cheese, *Bachman*	1 oz.	110	1½ B
Dutch,			
Mr. Salty	2 pretzels	104	1½ B
Rokeach	1 oz.	110	1½ B
Rokeach No-Salt	1 oz.	110	1½ B
Rods, *Seyfert's*	1 oz.	110	1½ B
Sticks, *Mr. Salty*	66 pieces	73	1 B
Sesame,			
and Bran sticks, *Flavor Tree*	1 oz.	160	1 B, 2 F
Chips, *Flavor Tree*	1 oz.	160	1 B, 2 F
Sticks, *Flavor Tree,*	1 oz.	160	1 B, 2 F
No-Salt	1 oz.	160	1 B, 2 F
Sour cream and onion	1 oz.	150	1 B, 2 F
Tortilla chips,			
Bachman	1 oz.	140	1 B, 1½ F
Cheese flavor, *Borden Lite-line*	1 oz.	130	1½ B, 1 F
Nacho cheese,			
Bachman	1 oz.	140	1 B, 1½ F
Buenos	14 chips	150	1 B, 1½ F
Nabisco	11 chips	125	1 B, 1 F
Wise Bravos	1 oz.	150	1 B, 1½ F
Sour cream and onion, *Buenos*	13 chips	140	1 B, 1½ F
Taco, *Bachman*	1 oz.	140	1 B, 1½ F

COOKIES AND BARS

Almond toast, *Stella D'Oro**	1 piece	56	1 B

*Contains sugar.

Product Name	Serving Size	Calories	Exchanges
Almond windmill, *Nabisco* *	2 cookies	95	1 B, ½ F
Angel bars, *Stella D'Oro* *	1 cookie	69	½ B, 1 F
Angel wings, *Stella D'Oro* *	1 cookie	75	½ B, 1 F
Anisette sponge, *Stella D'Oro* *	1 piece	52	1 B
Anisette toast, *Stella D'Oro* *	1 piece	46	½ B
Arrowroot biscuit, *National* *	4 cookies	87	1 B, ½ F
Bordeaux, *Pepperidge Farm Distinctive* *	3 cookies	110	1 B, 1 F
Brown Edge Wafers, *Nabisco* *	4 cookies	110	1 B, 1 F
Brownie chocolate nut, *Pepperidge Farm* *	3 cookies	170	1 B, 2½ F
Butter flavored, *Nabisco* *	4 cookies	93	1 B, ½ F
Chessmen, *Pepperidge Farm Distinctive* *	3 cookies	130	1 B, 1½ F
Chocolate chip,			
Nabisco Chips Ahoy *	2 cookies	105	1 B, 1 F
Pepperidge Farm *	3 cookies	150	1 B, 2 F
Chocolate wafers, *Nabisco* *	3 cookies	84	1 B, ½ F
Cinnamon sugar, *Pepperidge Farm* *	3 cookies	160	1 B, 2 F
Coconut granola, *Pepperidge Farm* *	3 cookies	170	1 B, 2½ F
Date nut granola, *Pepperidge Farm* *	3 cookies	160	1 B, 2 F
Egg biscuits, *Stella D'Oro* *	1 piece	44	½ B
Egg Jumbo, *Stella D'Oro* *	1 piece	46	½ B
Fig bars,			
Fig Newtons *	2 cookies	115	1 B, 1 F
Fig Wheats *	2 cookies	120	1½ B, ½ F
Fruit crescents, *Stella D'Oro* *	1 piece	55	1 B
Gingermen, *Pepperidge Farm Old Fashioned* *	3 cookies	100	1 B, 1 F
Ginger snaps, *Nabisco Old Fashioned* *	3 cookies	87	1 B, ½ F
Granola bars,			
Nature Valley, *			
Almond	1 bar	110	1 B, 1 F
Cinnamon	1 bar	110	1 B, 1 F
Coconut	1 bar	120	1 B, 1 F
Oats and honey	1 bar	110	1 B, 1 F
Peanut	1 bar	120	1 B, 1 F
Quaker, chewy, *			
Chocolate chip	1 bar	130	1½ B, 1 F
Honey and oats	1 bar	130	1½ B, 1 F

*Contains sugar.

Product Name	Serving Size	Calories	Exchanges
Peanut butter	1 bar	130	1½ B, 1 F
Raisin and cinnamon	1 bar	130	1½ B, 1 F
Lemon nut crunch, *Pepperidge Farm**	3 cookies	170	1 B, 2½ F
Margherite, *Stella D'Oro,**			
Chocolate	1 cookie	72	½ B, 1 F
Vanilla	1 cookie	75	½ B, 1 F
Molasses crisps, *Pepperidge Farm Old Fashioned**	3 cookies	100	1 B, 1 F
Oatmeal, Irish, *Pepperidge Farm Old Fashioned**	3 cookies	140	1½ B, 1 F
Orleans, *Pepperidge Farm Distinctive**	3 cookies	90	½ B, 1½ F
Peanut butter chip, *Pepperidge Farm Old Fashioned**	3 cookies	160	1 B, 2 F
Raisin bran, *Pepperidge Farm**	3 cookies	160	1 B, 2 F
Sesame, *Stella D'Oro**	1 piece	48	½ B
Shortbread,			
Lorna Doone*	3 cookies	118	1 B, 1 F
Pepperidge Farm Old Fashioned*	2 cookies	150	1 B, 1½ F
Sugar, *Pepperidge Farm**	3 cookies	150	1 B, 2 F
Sunflower raisin, *Pepperidge Farm**	3 cookies	160	1 B, 2 F
Vanilla wafers, *Nilla**	5 cookies	90	1 B, ½ F
Zanzibar, *Pepperidge Farm**	3 cookies	120	1 B, 1 F

CRACKERS

Product Name	Serving Size	Calories	Exchanges
Animal, *Ralston*	15 crackers	120	1½ B, ½ F
Biscuit,			
Social Tea	4 crackers	85	1 B, ½ F
Uneeda	4 crackers	87	1 B, ½ F
Butter flavored,			
Escort	6 crackers	130	1 B, 1½ F
Pepperidge Farm Goldfish Thins	8 crackers	70	1 B
Rich and Crisp	10 crackers	140	1½ B, 1 F
Ritz	8 crackers	133	1 B, 1½ F
Cheese,			
Cheez-it	14 pieces	80	½ B, 1 F
Nabisco,			
Cheddar Triangles	17 crackers	150	1 B, 1½ F
Swiss Cheese Flavored	13 crackers	126	1 B, 1½ F

*Contains sugar.

Product Name	Serving Size	Calories	Exchanges
Nips	23 crackers	116	1 B, 1 F
Pepperidge Farm,			
Goldfish Thins	8 crackers	80	½ B, 1 F
Snack Sticks	8 crackers	140	1½ B, 1 F
Snack Sticks, **Parmesan Pretzel**	8 crackers	120	1½ B, ½ F
Tiny Goldfish, **Cheddar**	45 crackers	140	1½ B, 1 F
Tiny Goldfish, **Parmesan**	45 crackers	140	1½ B, 1 F
Ralston	25 crackers	140	1½ B, 1 F
Rokeach	25 crackers	140	1 B, 1½ F
Tid-Bit	32 crackers	149	1 B, 2 F
Cheese sandwich,			
Nabisco Nab Pack	4 pieces	118	1 B, 1 F
Crispbread, *RyKrisp,*			
Natural	2 triple crackers	50	½ B
Seasoned	2 triple crackers	60	1 B
Sesame	2 triple crackers	60	1 B
Graham,			
Honey Maid	3 crackers	89	1 B, ½ F
Nabisco	3 crackers	89	1 B, ½ F
Cinnamon Treats	3 crackers	81	1 B, ½ F
Ralston	8 crackers	120	1½ B, ½ F
Rokeach	8 crackers	120	1½ B, ½ F
Matzos, *Manischewitz,*			
American	1 matzo	115	1½ B
Crackers	5 crackers	45	½ B
Egg n' Onion	1 matzo	112	1½ B
Egg, for Passover	1 matzo	132	2 B
Passover.	1 matzo	129	2 B
Thins	1 matzo	91	1½ B
Thin, salted	1 matzo	95	1½ B
Thin Tea,	1 matzo	103	1½ B
for Passover	1 matzo	103	1½ B
Unsalted	1 matzo	112	1½ B
Whole wheat with bran	1 matzo	110	1½ B
Whole wheat for Passover	1 matzo	118	1½ B
Melba toast,			
Lance	2 slices	37	½ B
Old London,			
Bacon Rounds	5 crackers	60	½ B, ½ F
Cheese Rounds	5 crackers	60	½ B, ½ F
Garlic Rounds	5 crackers	50	½ B

Product Name	Serving Size	Calories	Exchanges
Onion Rounds	5 crackers	50	½ B
Pumpernickel	3 slices	50	½ B
Rye	3 slices	50	½ B
Salty Rye Rounds	5 crackers	50	½ B
Sesame Rounds	5 crackers	60	½ B, ½ F
White	3 slices	50	½ B
Whole grain	3 slices	60	1 B
Milk, *Royal Lunch*	2 crackers	106	1 B, 1 F
Oyster,			
Dandy	30 crackers	87	1 B, ½ F
Oysterettes	27 crackers	85	1 B, ½ F
Ralston	33 crackers	120	1½ B, ½ F
Sunshine	18 crackers	70	1 B
Peanut butter sandwich,			
Nekot	1 pkg. (1½ oz.)	208	1½ B, ½ M, 1½ F
Nip-Chee	1 pkg. (1¼ oz.)	183	1 B, ½ M, 2 F
Toastchee	1 pkg. (1⅜ oz.)	198	1 B, ½ M, 2 F
Cheese,			
Keebler	6 pieces	210	2 B, 1½ F
Nabisco Nab Pack	4 pieces	135	1 B, 1½ F
Malt, *Lance*	1 pkg. (1¼ oz.)	187	1 B, ½ M, 2 F
Malted milk, *Nabisco Nab Pack*	4 pieces	138	1 B, 1½ F
Toast,			
Keebler	6 pieces	230	2 B, 2 F
Lance	1 pkg. (1¼ oz.)	180	1 B, ½ M, 1½ F
Pizza flavored, *Pepperidge Farm Tiny Goldfish*	45 pieces	140	1 B, 1½ F
Pretzel, *Pepperidge Farm Tiny Goldfish*	40 pieces	120	1½ B, ½ F
Pumpernickel, *Pepperidge Farm Snack Sticks*	8 crackers	130	1½ B, ½ F
Rusk, *Holland*	2 crackers	82	1 B, ½ F
Rye,			
Lance Rye Twins	2 crackers	32	½ B
Pepperidge Farm Snack Sticks	8 crackers	130	1½ B, ½ F
Salted, *Pepperidge Farm,*			
Goldfish Thins	8 crackers	80	½ B, 1 F
Snack Sticks	8 crackers	130	1½ B, ½ F
Tiny Goldfish	45 crackers	140	1 B, 1½ F
Saltines,			
Lance	4 crackers	49	½ B
Premium,	7 crackers	82	1 B, ½ F

Product Name	Serving Size	Calories	Exchanges
Unsalted tops	7 crackers	85	1 B, ½ F
Ralston,	10 crackers	120	1½ B, ½ F
Unsalted tops	10 crackers	120	1½ B, ½ F
Rokeach	10 crackers	120	1½ B, ½ F
Sunshine Krispy	4 crackers	50	½ B
Sesame,			
Lance	2 crackers	40	½ B
Nabisco,			
Meal Mates	5 crackers	108	1 B, 1 F
Sesame Snack	8 crackers	131	1 B, 1½ F
Pepperidge Farm,			
Distinctive	6 crackers	140	1 B, 1½ F
Snack Sticks	8 crackers	130	1 B, 1½ F
Sesame Wheats	9 crackers	150	1 B, 2 F
Sesame/Cheese Twigs	10 pieces	138	1 B, 1½ F
Snack,			
Bacon Flavored Thins, *Nabisco*	12 crackers	128	1 B, 1½ F
French Onion, *Nabisco*	10 crackers	121	1 B, 1 F
Garlic Tams	5 crackers	65	½ B, ½ F
Onion Tams	5 crackers	65	½ B, ½ F
Rokeach	9 crackers	130	1 B, 1½ F
Snack Shapes	15 crackers	140	1 B, 1½ F
Snackers	8 crackers	140	1 B, 1½ F
Sociables	11 crackers	117	1 B, 1 F
Tam Tams	5 crackers	70	½ B, ½ F
Vegetable Thins, *Nabisco*	13 crackers	150	1 B, 1½ F
Soda,			
Captain's Wafers	2 crackers	32	½ B
Crown Pilot	1 cracker	72	1 B
Gitana	6 crackers	86	1 B, ½ F
Sea Rounds	2 crackers	89	1 B, ½ F
Unsalted, *Estee*	2 crackers	30	½ B
Water biscuit, English,			
Pepperidge Farm Distinctive	7 crackers	120	1½ B, ½ F
Wheat,			
Featherweight,			
Unsalted wafers	4 wafers	50	½ B
Unsalted bran wafers	4 wafers	50	½ B
Manischewitz	5 crackers	45	½ B
Pepperidge Farm Goldfish Thins	8 crackers	80	½ B, ½ F
Ralston	15 crackers	140	1½ B, 1 F

Product Name	Serving Size	Calories	Exchanges
Triscuit Wafers	5 crackers	102	1 B, 1 F
Wheat Thins	13 crackers	112	1 B, 1 F
Wheatsworth	9 crackers	130	1 B, 1½ F
Cracked, *Pepperidge Farm Distinctive*	5 crackers	140	1 B, 1½ F
Hearty, *Pepperidge Farm Distinctive*	5 crackers	140	1 B, 1½ F
Wheatgerm wafers, *Estee*	10 crackers	36	½ B
Zwieback, *Nabisco*	3 pieces	93	1 B, ½ F

CROUTONS, CRUMBS, AND CRUSTS

Product Name	Serving Size	Calories	Exchanges
Bread crumbs,			
Regular, *Old London*	1 tbsp.	50	1 B
Seasoned, *Contadina*	1 tbsp.	35	½ B
Croutons,			
All flavors, *Salad Crispins*	1 tsp.	14	free in moderation
Buttery, *Brownberry*	1 oz.	130	1½ B, ½ F
Caesar salad, *Brownberry*	1 oz.	130	1½ B, ½ F
Cheddar cheese, *Brownberry*	1 oz.	130	1½ B, ½ F
Cheddar and romano cheese, *Pepperidge Farm*	½ oz.	60	1 B
Cheese and garlic, *Pepperidge Farm*	½ oz.	70	1 B
Onion and garlic,			
Brownberry	1 oz.	130	1½ B, ½ F
Pepperidge Farm	½ oz.	70	1 B
Ranch style, *Brownberry*	1 oz.	130	1½ B, ½ F
Seasoned,			
Brownberry	1 oz.	130	1½ B, ½ F
Pepperidge Farm	½ oz.	70	1 B
Sexton cheese, *Brownberry*	1 oz.	130	1½ B, ½ F
Sour cream and chive, *Pepperidge Farm*	½ oz.	70	1 B
Toasted, *Brownberry*	1 oz.	120	1½ B, ½ F
Patty shells, *Pepperidge Farm*	1 shell	210	1 B, 3 F
Pie crust,			
Pillsbury All-Ready	⅛ of 2-crust pie	240	1½ B, 3 F
Mix,			
Flako	⅙ of 9-inch crust	260	2 B, 2½ F
General Mills	1/16 pkg.	120	1 B, 1 F
General Mills, stick	⅛ stick	110	½ B, 1½ F
Pillsbury	⅙ pie	270	1½ B, 3½ F

Product Name	Serving Size	Calories	Exchanges
Puff pastry sheets, *Pepperidge Farm*	1 sheet	510	3 B, 7 F

PANCAKES, WAFFLES, AND FRENCH TOAST

French toast, frozen,
Aunt Jemima,	2 slices	170	2 B, 1 F
Cinnamon Swirl	2 slices	210	2 B, 1½ F

Pancake batter,
Aunt Jemima	three 4″ pancakes	210	3 B
Pillsbury Panshakes	three 4″ pancakes	250	3 B, 1 F

Pancake mix,
Dia-Mel	three 4″ pancakes	100	1½ B
Featherweight	three 4″ pancakes	130	2 B
Hungry Jack Extra Lights	three 4″ pancakes	200	2 B, 1½ F
Pillsbury Golden Blend,	three 4″ pancakes	200	2 B, 1½ F
Complete	three 4″ pancakes	240	3 B, 1 F

Blueberry,
Aunt Jemima	three 4″ pancakes	210	3 B
Pillsbury	three 4″ pancakes	320	2 B, 3 F, 1 Fr

Buttermilk,
Aunt Jemima	three 4″ pancakes	210	3 B
Hungry Jack	three 4″ pancakes	240	2 B, 2 F
Pillsbury **Complete**	three 4″ pancakes	190	2½ B, ½ F

Pancake and waffle mix,
Aunt Jemima,	three 4″ pancakes	220	2 B, 1½ F
Complete	three 4″ pancakes	240	3 B, 1 F

Buttermilk,
Aunt Jemima	three 4″ pancakes	300	3 B, ½ M, 1½ F
Aunt Jemima **Complete**	three 4″ pancakes	240	3 B, 1 F
General Mills	⅓ cup prepared	280	2½ B, 2½ F
Buckwheat, *Aunt Jemima*	three 4″ pancakes	200	2 B, 1½ F
Whole wheat, *Aunt Jemima*	three 4″ pancakes	250	2 B, ½ M, 2 F

Waffles, frozen,
Aunt Jemima Jumbo,	1 waffle	80	1 B, ½ F
Apple and Cinnamon	1 waffle	80	1 B, ½ F
Blueberry	1 waffle	80	1 B, ½ F
Buttermilk	1 waffle	80	1 B, ½ F

PASTA

All shapes of plain pasta made by each manufacturer have the same nutrient content, calories, and exchanges. Similarly, all egg pasta products are the same for each manufacturer. Plain pasta shapes include linguine, macaroni, lasagna, spaghetti, shells, and vermicelli. Egg pasta shapes include egg noodles, egg bows, egg pastina, and fettucine. High-protein pasta has approximately the same number of calories per serving as regular pasta, but contains more protein and less carbohydrate.

"Light" pasta absorbs more water during cooking than regular pasta, thus increasing more in bulk. It has the same number of calories as regular pasta on a "dry weight" basis, but one-third fewer calories on a "cooked weight" basis. Prepared pastas listed here are side dishes—noodles with sauces or seasonings. Canned and frozen pasta dishes and macaroni mixes are listed in Chapter 1, under COMBINATION MAIN DISHES.

Product Name	Serving Size	Calories	Exchanges
Egg pasta,			
American Beauty	2 oz. dry	220	2½ B, ½ M, ½ F
Creamette	2 oz. dry	220	2½ B, ½ M, ½ F
Pennsylvania Dutch	2 oz. dry	210	2½ B, ½ M, ½ F
Ronzoni	2 oz. dry	220	2½ B, ½ M, ½ F
High-protein pasta,			
Prince Superoni	2 oz. dry	204	2 B, 1 M
"Light" pasta,			
Prince Light	1.4 oz. dry	140	2 B
Plain pasta,			
American Beauty	2 oz. dry	200	3 B
Creamette	2 oz. dry	210	3 B
Prince	2 oz. dry	204	3 B
Ronzoni	2 oz. dry	210	3 B
Spinach pasta, *Creamette*	2 oz. dry	200	3 B
Prepared pasta,			
Chow mein noodles, *La Choy*	½ cup	150	1 B, 1½ F
Egg noodles,			
and Beef flavor sauce, *Lipton*	½ cup prepared	190	2 B, 1 F
and Butter sauce, *Lipton*	½ cup prepared	190	1½ B, 2 F
and Butter and herb sauce, *Lipton*	½ cup prepared	180	1½ B, 1½ F
and Cheese sauce, *Lipton*	½ cup prepared	200	1½ B, ½ M, 1½ F
and Chicken flavor sauce, *Lipton*	½ cup prepared	190	1½ B, 2 F
and Sour cream and chive sauce, *Lipton*	½ cup prepared	190	1½ B, 2 F

Product Name	Serving Size	Calories	Exchanges
Fettucini Alfredo, frozen, *Stouffer's*	5.0 oz.	270	1½ B, ½ M, 3 F
Noodles,			
Almondine, *General Mills*	¼ pkg. prepared	240	1½ B, ½ M, 2½ F
Parmesan, *Golden Grain Noodle Roni Parmesano*	½ cup prepared	130	1½ B, ½ M
Romanoff, *General Mills*	¼ pkg. prepared	230	1½ B, ½ M, 2 F
Romanoff, frozen, *Stouffer's*	4.0 oz.	170	1 B, ½ M, 1½ F
Stroganoff, *General Mills*	¼ pkg. prepared	240	1½ B, ½ M, 2½ F
Rice noodles, *La Choy*	½ cup	130	1½ B, ½ F

RICE

Product Name	Serving Size	Calories	Exchanges
Plain,			
Brown, parboiled, *Uncle Ben's*	⅔ cup prepared	152	1½ B, 1 F
White,			
Minute	⅔ cup prepared	120	1½ B
Uncle Ben's Converted	⅔ cup prepared	148	2 B
Uncle Ben's Quick	⅔ cup prepared	143	2 B
Prepared,			
Beef flavored mix,			
Golden Grain Rice-A-Roni	½ cup prepared	130	2 B
Minute Rib Roast	½ cup prepared	150	1½ B, 1 F
Brown and wild seasoned mix, *Uncle Ben's*	½ cup prepared	150	1½ B, 1 F
Chicken flavored mix,			
Golden Grain Rice-A-Roni	¾ cup prepared	160	2½ B
Minute Drumstick	½ cup prepared	150	1½ B, 1 F
Country French Style, frozen, *Rice Originals*	½ cup	160	1½ B, 1 F
Festive Rice, frozen, *Rice Originals*	½ cup	140	1½ B, 1 F
French Style, frozen, *Birds Eye*	3.6 oz.	120	2 B
Fried rice,			
Canned, *La Choy*	¾ cup	190	2½ B, ½ F
Frozen, *Birds Eye*	3.6 oz.	110	1½ B
Mix, *Durkee*	½ cup prepared	108	1½ B
Mix, *Minute*	½ cup prepared	160	1½ B, 1 F
Italian Style, frozen, *Birds Eye*	3.6 oz.	130	2 B
Long grain and wild rice, mix,			
Minute	½ cup prepared	150	1½ B, 1 F
Uncle Ben's	½ cup prepared	113	1½ B
Uncle Ben's fast-cooking	½ cup prepared	127	1½ B, ½ F

Product Name	Serving Size	Calories	Exchanges
Northern Italian Style, frozen, *Birds Eye*	3.6 oz.	110	1½ B
Oriental Style, frozen, *Birds Eye*	3.6 oz.	130	2 B
Rice and broccoli in cheese sauce, frozen, *Rice Originals*	½ cup	140	1 B, ½ V, 1 F
Rice with herb butter sauce, frozen, *Rice Originals*	½ cup	150	1½ B, 1 F
Rice Medley, frozen, *Rice Originals*	½ cup	120	1½ B, ½ F
Rice and peas with mushrooms, frozen, *Birds Eye*	2.3 oz.	110	1½ B
Rice pilaf, frozen, *Rice Originals*	½ cup	120	1½ B, ½ F
Rice and spinach in cheese sauce, Italian, frozen, *Rice Originals*	½ cup	160	1½ B, 1½ F
Rice Verdi, frozen, *Rice Originals*	½ cup	130	1½ B, ½ F
Spanish,			
Canned, *Van Camp*	8 oz.	160	1½ B, 1F
Frozen, *Birds Eye*	3.6 oz.	120	2 B
Mix, *Golden Grain Rice-A-Roni*	¾ cup prepared	120	1½ B
Mix, *Minute*	½ cup prepared	150	1½ B, 1 F
White and wild rice, frozen, *Rice Originals*	½ cup	110	1½ B

STUFFING

Brownberry, all flavors	½ cup prepared	170	1½ B, 1½ F
Pepperidge Farm, all flavors	1 oz. dry	110	1½ B
Stove Top,			
Beef	½ cup prepared	180	1½ B, 1½ F
Chicken flavor	½ cup prepared	170	1½ B, 1½ F
Cornbread	½ cup prepared	170	1½ B, 1½ F
New England Style	½ cup prepared	180	1½ B, 1½ F
Pork	½ cup prepared	170	1½ B, 1½ F
with Rice	½ cup prepared	180	1½ B, 1½ F
San Francisco Style	½ cup prepared	170	1½ B, 1½ F

6

SOUPS

☐ Condensed and
undiluted canned

☐ Frozen

☐ Instant and cooked mixes

Commercially packaged soups are convenient, quick, and tasty. Broths and bouillons, both canned and instant, can be used alone, as the base for a more complex soup, or as a seasoning for gravies, sauces, and stews. Low in calories (most are free in moderation), broths and bouillons are also useful during sick days as an easy-to-digest way to replace lost fluids and salt. Cream soups and chowders are higher in calories, but still provide good nutrition.

Many, such as cream of mushroom, tomato, or onion, can also be used in gravies or sauces. If you do use soups as ingredients in other foods, remember to work the exchanges into your meal plan.

We've broken the soups listed here into five groups—canned condensed, canned undiluted, frozen, cooked mixes, and instant mixes. All serving sizes are listed as *prepared ounces*, using the amount of liquid called for in the package directions. Unless otherwise noted, exchanges for all condensed soups are calculated as diluted with water. Some mixes require the addition of meat; we calculated exchanges to include the added meat.

Undiluted soups are measured straight

from the can, while mixes and condensed soups are measured *after* adding the appropriate amount of liquid. Eight ounces (by weight) is the most common serving size for condensed soups. The easiest way to measure your portion is to look on the label to find out how many eight-ounce servings the can will make. Divide the prepared soup by that number of servings to get the appropriate serving size. Soup mix serving sizes vary, but you can use the same procedure to determine them. Or, since mixes are measured in fluid ounces (fl. oz.), you can use a measuring cup to find your portion. (To convert fluid ounces into cups, see Appendix I.)

Because they're a blend of many ingredients, some soups will include several exchange groups. If you eat more or less than the serving size listed here, remember to adjust *all* the exchanges accordingly.

Product Name	Serving Size	Calories	Exchanges

CANNED

■ Condensed

Product Name	Serving Size	Calories	Exchanges
Asparagus, cream of, *Campbell's*	8 oz.	90	1 B, ½ F
Bean,			
with Bacon, *Campbell's*	8 oz.	150	1½ B, 1 F
Black, *Campbell's*	8 oz.	110	1 B, ½ M
Old-fashioned, with ham, *Campbell's Soup for One*	11 oz.	220	2 B, ½ M, 1 F
Beef,			
Campbell's	8 oz.	80	1 B, ½ M
Broth,			
Campbell's	8 oz.	15	free in moderation
and Barley, *Campbell's*	8 oz.	60	½ B, ½ F
and Noodles, *Campbell's*	8 oz.	60	½ B, ½ F
Noodle, *Campbell's*	8 oz.	70	½ B, ½ M
Teriyaki, *Campbell's*	8 oz.	70	½ B, ½ M
Celery, cream of,			
Campbell's	8 oz.	100	½ B, 1½ F
Rokeach	10 oz.*	190	½ B, 1½ F, 1 Mk
Cheddar cheese, *Campbell's*	8 oz.	130	½ B, ½ M, 1½ F
Chicken,			
Alphabet, *Campbell's*	8 oz.	80	½ B, ½ M, ½ F
Broth,			
Campbell's	4 oz.	17	free in moderation
and Noodles, *Campbell's*	8 oz.	60	½ B, ½ F

*Prepared with whole milk.

Product Name	Serving Size	Calories	Exchanges
and Rice, *Campbell's*	8 oz.	50	½ B, ½ F
and Vegetables, *Campbell's*	8 oz.	25	1 V
Cream of, *Campbell's*	8 oz.	110	½ B, ½ M, 1 F
and Dumplings, *Campbell's*	8 oz.	90	½ B, ½ M, ½ F
Gumbo, *Campbell's*	8 oz.	60	½ B, ½ F
Mushroom, creamy, *Campbell's*	8 oz.	110	½ B, ½ M, 1 F
Noodle,			
Campbell's	8 oz.	70	½ B, ½ M
Featherweight	7¼ oz.	60	½ B, ½ M
Golden, *Campbell's* Soup for One	11 oz.	130	1 B, ½ M, ½ F
NoodleO's, Campbell's	8 oz.	70	½ B, ½ F
Oriental, *Campbell's*	8 oz.	50	½ B, ½ F
with Rice, *Campbell's*	8 oz.	60	½ B, ½ F
and Stars, *Campbell's*	8 oz.	60	½ B, ½ F
Vegetable,			
Campbell's	8 oz.	70	½ B, ½ F
Campbell's Soup for One	11 oz.	120	1 B, 1 F
Chili beef, *Campbell's*	8 oz.	130	1 B, ½ M, ½ F
Clam chowder,			
Manhattan,			
Campbell's	8 oz.	70	½ B, ½ F, ½ V
Snow's	7½ oz.	70	½ B, ½ F, ½ V
New England,			
Campbell's	8 oz.*	165	1 B, ½ M, ½ F, ½ Mk
Campbell's Soup for One	11 oz.*	200	1 B, ½ M, 1½ F, ½ Mk
Snow's	7½ oz.*	140	½ B, ½ M, 1 F, ½ Mk
Consommé, beef, *Campbell's*	4 oz.	13	free in moderation
Corn chowder, New England, *Snow's*	7½ oz.*	150	½ B, 1½ F, ½ Mk
Fish chowder, New England, *Snow's*	7½ oz.*	130	½ B, ½ M, ½ F, ½ Mk
Meatball alphabet, *Campbell's*	8 oz.	100	1 B, ½ M
Minestrone, *Campbell's*	8 oz.	80	½ B, ½ F, ½ V
Mushroom,			
Barley, *Campbell's*	8 oz.	80	1 B, ½ F
Beefy, *Campbell's*	8 oz.	70	½ B, ½ M
Cream of,			
Campbell's	8 oz.	100	½ B, 1½ F
Campbell's Soup for One	11 oz.	180	1 B, 2½ F

*Prepared with whole milk.

Product Name	Serving Size	Calories	Exchanges
Featherweight	7¼ oz.	50	½ B, ½ F
Rokeach	10 oz.*	240	½ B, 3 F, 1 Mk
Golden, Campbell's	8 oz.	80	1 B, ½ F
Noodle,			
Curly, with chicken, Campbell's	8 oz.	70	½ B, ½ F
and ground beef, Campbell's	8 oz.	90	½ B, ½ M, ½ F
Onion,			
Campbell's	8 oz.**	145	1 B, 1 F, ½ Mk
French, Campbell's	8 oz.	70	½ B, ½ F
Oyster stew, Campbell's	8 oz.**	155	½ B, 1½ F, ½ Mk
Pea,			
Green, Campbell's	8 oz.	150	2 B, ½ F
Split, with ham and bacon, Campbell's	8 oz.	170	1½ B, ½ M, ½ F
Pepper pot, Campbell's	8 oz.	90	½ B, ½ M, ½ F
Potato, cream of, Campbell's	8 oz.**	115	½ B, 1 F, ½ Mk
Scotch broth, Campbell's	8 oz.	80	½ B, ½ M, ½ F
Seafood chowder, New England, Snow's	7½ oz.*	130	½ B, ½ M, ½ F, ½ Mk
Shrimp, cream of, Campbell's	8 oz.*	175	½ B, 2 F, ½ Mk
Tomato,			
Campbell's	8 oz.	90	½ B, ½ F, ½ V
Featherweight	8 oz.	60	½ B, 1 V
Rokeach	10 oz.	90	½ B, 2 V
Bisque, Campbell's	8 oz.	120	1 B, ½ F, ½ V
Garden, Campbell's	8 oz.	80	½ B, 1½ V
Rice,			
Rokeach	10 oz.	160	1 B, 1 F, 1½ V
Old-fashioned, Campbell's	8 oz.	110	1 B, ½ F, ½ V
Royale, Campbell's Soup for One	11 oz.	180	1½ B, 1 F, ½ V
Turkey,			
Noodle, Campbell's	8 oz.	60	½ B, ½ F
Vegetable, Campbell's	8 oz.	70	½ B, ½ F
Vegetable,			
Campbell's	8 oz.	80	½ B, ½ F, ½ V
Beef,			
Campbell's	8 oz.	70	½ B, ½ F
Featherweight	7¼ oz.	80	½ B, ½ F, ½ V

*Prepared with whole milk.
**Prepared with whole milk and water.

Product Name	Serving Size	Calories	Exchanges

Burly, *Campbell's*
Soup for One . . . . 11 oz. . . . . 150 . . . . 1 B, ½ M, ½ F, 1 V

Old-fashioned, *Campbell's* . . . . . . 8 oz. . . . . 60 . . . . ½ B, 1 V

Old World, *Campbell's*
Soup for One . . . . 11 oz. . . . . 130 . . . . 1 B, 1 F, 1 V

Spanish style
(gazpacho), *Campbell's* . . . . 8 oz. . . . . 50 . . . . ½ B, 1 V

Vegetarian,
Campbell's . . . . 8 oz. . . . . 70 . . . . ½ B, ½ F, ½ V
Rokeach . . . . 10 oz. . . . . 90 . . . . ½ B, ½ F, 1 V

Won ton, *Campbell's* . . . . 8 oz. . . . . 40 . . . . ½ B

■ Undiluted

Bean with ham, chunky old-fashioned,
Campbell's . . . . 9½ oz. . . . . 250 . . . . 2 B, 1 M, 1½ F
Campbell's Individual Size . . . . 11 oz. . . . . 290 . . . . 2 B, 1½ M, 1½ F

Beef,
Broth, *Swanson* . . . . 7¼ oz. . . . . 20 . . . . . . free in moderation

Chunky,
Campbell's . . . . 9½ oz. . . . . 170 . . . . 1 B, 1 M, 1 F
Campbell's Individual Size . . . . . 10¾ oz. . . . . 190 . . . . 1½ B, 1 M, ½ F

and Mushroom, low sodium,
chunky, *Campbell's* . . . . 10¾ oz. . . . . 200 . . . . 1½ B, 1 M, 1 F

with Noodles, chunky,
Campbell's Individual Size . . . . . . 10¾ oz. . . . . 300 . . . . 2 B, 1½ M, 2 F

Chicken,
Broth, *Swanson* . . . . 4 oz. . . . . 20 . . . . . . free in moderation

Chunky,
Campbell's . . . . 9½ oz. . . . . 180 . . . . 1½ B, 1½ M
Campbell's Individual Size . . . . . 10¾ oz. . . . . 210 . . . . 1½ B, 1½ M, ½ F
Low sodium, *Campbell's* . . . . . . 7½ oz. . . . . 150 . . . . 1 B, 1 M, ½ F

Noodle,
Dia-Mel . . . . 8 oz. . . . . 50 . . . . ½ B, ½ M
Low sodium, *Campbell's* . . . . . . 7¼ oz. . . . . 90 . . . . ½ B, ½ M, ½ F

Low sodium, *Campbell's*
Individual Size . . . . 10¾ oz. . . . . 180 . . . . 1 B, 1½ M, ½ F

with Rice, chunky, *Campbell's* . . . . 9½ oz. . . . . 140 . . . . 1 B, 1 M, ½ F

Vegetable, chunky,
Campbell's . . . . 9½ oz. . . . . 170 . . . . 1 B, 1 M, ½ F, ½ V
Low sodium, *Campbell's* . . . . . . 10¾ oz. . . . . 240 . . . . . . 1 B, 1½ M, 1½ F, 1 V

Chili beef, chunky,
Campbell's . . . . 9¾ oz. . . . . 260 . . . . 2 B, 2 M
Campbell's Individual Size . . . . 11 oz. . . . . 300 . . . . 2½ B, 2½ M

Product Name	Serving Size	Calories	Exchanges
Clam chowder, Manhattan, chunky, *Campbell's*	9½ oz.	150	1 B, ½ M, ½ F, 1 V
Ham and butter bean, chunky, *Campbell's Individual Size*	10¾ oz.	280	2 B, 1½ M, 1½ F
Minestrone, chunky, *Campbell's*	9½ oz.	150	1 B, 1 F, 1 V
Mushroom, cream of,			
Dia-Mel	8 oz.	85	1 F, ½ Mk
Low sodium, *Campbell's*	7¼ oz.	130	½ B, 2 F
Pea, split,			
with ham, chunky,			
Campbell's	9½ oz.	200	2 B, 1 M
Campbell's Individual Size	10¾ oz.	230	2 B, 1 M, 1 F
Low sodium, *Campbell's*	10¾ oz.	220	2 B, 1 M, ½ F
Sirloin burger, chunky,			
Campbell's	9½ oz.	200	1½ B, 1 M, 1 F
Campbell's Individual Size	10½ oz.	220	1½ B, 1½ M, 1 F
Steak and potato, chunky,			
Campbell's	9½ oz.	170	1½ B, 1 M, ½ F
Campbell's Individual Size	10¾ oz.	190	1½ B, 1½ M
Tomato,			
Dia-Mel	8 oz.	50	½ B, 1 V
Low sodium, *Campbell's*	7¼ oz.	140	1 B, ½ F, 1½ V
with tomato pieces, low sodium, *Campbell's*	10½ oz.	200	1½ B, 1 F, 2 V
Turkey,			
Chunky, *Campbell's*	9¼ oz.	180	1½ B, 1 M, ½ F
Noodle, low sodium, *Campbell's*	7¼ oz.	70	½ B, ½ M
Vegetable,			
Chunky,			
Campbell's	9½ oz.	130	1 B, ½ F, 1 V
Campbell's Individual Size	10¾ oz.	140	1 B, 1 F, 1 V
Low sodium, *Campbell's*	7¼ oz.	90	½ B, ½ F, 1 V
Mediterranean, chunky, *Campbell's*	9½ oz.	170	1½ B, 1 F, 1 V
Three-bean, chunky, *Campbell's*	9½ oz.	210	2 B, 1 F, 1 V
Vegetable beef,			
Dia-Mel	8 oz.	70	½ B, ½ F, ½ V
Chunky old-fashioned,			
Campbell's	9½ oz.	160	1 B, 1 M, 1 V
Campbell's Individual Size	10¾ oz.	180	1 B, 1 M, ½ F, 1 V
Low sodium,			
Campbell's	7¼ oz.	90	½ B, 1 M, ½ V

Product Name	Serving Size	Calories	Exchanges
Chunky, *Campbell's*	10¾ oz.	180	1 B, 1½ M, 1 V

FROZEN

Cream of spinach, *Stouffer's*	8 oz.	230	½ B, ½ V, 3 F, ½ Mk
New England clam chowder, *Stouffer's*	8 oz.	200	½ B, ½ M, 1½ F, 1 Mk
Split pea with ham, *Stouffer's*	8¼ oz.	190	2 B, 1 M

MIXES

■ Cooked

Beef,

Barley, *Homemade Soup Starter*	12 fl. oz.	275	2 B, 2 M, ½ F
Mushroom, *Lipton*	8 fl. oz.	40	½ B
Noodle, *Homemade Soup Starter*	12 fl. oz.	255	1½ B, 2 M, 1 F
Vegetable, *Homemade Soup Starter*	12 fl. oz.	275	2 B, 2 M, ½ F

Chicken,

Cream of, *Estee*	1 envelope	50	1 B
Noodle, *Homemade Soup Starter*	12 fl. oz.	255	1½ B, 2 M, 1 F
Rice, *Lipton*	8 fl. oz.	60	½ B, ½ M
Ripple noodle, *Lipton*	8 fl. oz.	80	1 B
Vegetable, *Homemade Soup Starter*	12 fl. oz.	265	1½ B, 2 M, 1 F

Ground beef vegetable, *Homemade Soup Starter*	12 fl. oz.	340	1½ B, 2½ M, 2 F
Minestrone, *Manischewitz*	6 fl. oz.	50	½ B, ½ V
Mushroom, cream of, *Estee*	1 envelope	50	1 B

Noodle,

Lipton Giggle	8 fl. oz.	80	1 B
Lipton Ring-O	8 fl. oz.	60	1 B

Onion,

Lipton	8 fl. oz.	35	½ B
Beefy, *Lipton*	8 fl. oz.	30	½ B
Mushroom, *Lipton*	8 fl. oz.	40	½ B

Pea, split, *Manischewitz*	6 fl. oz.	45	½ B

Tomato,

Cream of, *Estee*	1 envelope	60	½ B, ½ V
Vegetable, *Estee*	1 envelope	60	½ B, ½ V

Vegetable,

Manischewitz	6 fl. oz.	50	½ B, ½ V
Beef, *Lipton*	8 fl. oz.	50	½ B, ½ V

Product Name	Serving Size	Calories	Exchanges
Country, *Lipton*	8 fl. oz.	80	1 B, ½ V
Cream of, *Estee*	1 envelope	60	1 B

■Instant

Beef,

Bouillon,

Featherweight	1 tsp. (dry)	18	free in moderation
Wyler's	1 tsp. (dry)	6	free in moderation
Broth, *Weight Watchers*	1 packet	8	free in moderation

Flavor,

Lipton Lots-A-Noodles Cup-A-Soup	7 fl. oz.	120	1½ B, ½ F
Noodle, *Lipton Cup-A-Soup*	6 fl. oz.	50	1 B

Chicken,

Bouillon,

Featherweight	1 tsp. (dry)	18	free in moderation
Wyler's	1 cube	8	free in moderation

Broth,

Lipton Cup-A-Soup	6 fl. oz.	25	½ B
Weight Watchers	1 packet	8	free in moderation
Cream of, *Lipton Cup-A-Soup*	6 fl. oz.	80	½ B, 1 F
Flavor, *Lipton Lots-A-Noodles Cup-A-Soup*	7 fl. oz.	130	1½ B, ½ F
Hearty, *Country Style Cup-A-Soup*	6 fl. oz.	70	½ B, ½ M
Noodle with meat, *Lipton Cup-A-Soup*	6 fl. oz.	45	½ B
Rice, *Lipton Cup-A-Soup*	6 fl. oz.	45	½ B
Supreme, *Country Style Cup-A-Soup*	6 fl. oz.	100	1 B, 1 F
Vegetable, *Lipton Cup-A-Soup*	6 fl. oz.	40	½ B
Mushroom, cream of, *Lipton Cup-A-Soup*	6 fl. oz.	80	½ B, 1 F

Onion,

Lipton Cup-A-Soup	6 fl. oz.	30	½ B
Bouillon, *Wyler's*	1 tsp. (dry)	10	free in moderation
Broth, *Weight Watchers*	1 packet	8	free in moderation
Oriental style, *Lipton Lots-A-Noodles Cup-A-Soup*	7 fl. oz.	130	1½ B, ½ F

Pea,

Green, *Lipton Cup-A-Soup*	6 fl. oz.	120	1 B, 1 F
Virginia, *Country Style Cup-A-Soup*	6 fl. oz.	140	1 B, ½ M, 1 F

Product Name	Serving Size	Calories	Exchanges
Ring noodle, *Lipton Cup-A-Soup*	6 fl. oz.	50	1 B
Tomato, *Lipton Cup-A-Soup*	6 fl. oz.	80	1 B, ½ V
Vegetable,			
Beef, *Lipton Cup-A-Soup*	6 fl. oz.	50	½ B, ½ V
Garden, *Lipton Lots-A-Noodles Cup-A-Soup*	7 fl. oz.	130	1½ B, ½ F
Harvest, *Country Style Cup-A-Soup*	6 fl. oz.	100	1½ B
Spring, *Lipton Cup-A-Soup*	6 fl. oz.	40	½ B

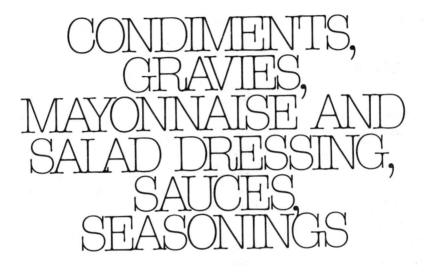

7

CONDIMENTS, GRAVIES, MAYONNAISE, AND SALAD DRESSING, SAUCES, SEASONINGS

In this chapter you'll find catsup, pickles, mustard, mayonnaise, gravies, marinades, spaghetti sauces, salad dressings, spices, and lots of other items to add flavor and variety to your meals. Many condiments and seasonings are free exchanges or free in moderation. Some of the seasonings listed are flavoring mixes for main dishes, such as stew or tacos. Exchanges for these are for the seasoning *alone*, because we couldn't determine values for the prepared dishes. (For other main-dish seasonings calculated in prepared form, see Chapter 1 under COMBINATION MAIN DISHES —Mixes.)

Gravies and sauces vary considerably in calories and exchange values, depending on variety and brand. Many mixes made with water are free in moderation. Bottled and canned gravies are higher in fat and may count as fat exchanges, while spaghetti and pizza sauces are usually a combination of bread, fat, and vegetable exchanges.

Regular salad dressings and mayonnaises are high in calories—just one tablespoon of many varieties equals one or more fat exchanges. But for those days when you want to use your fat exchanges in other ways, "diet" dressings are listed as well. Most imitation mayonnaises are low in oil and have only about one-third the calories of the regular kind. Diet or low-calorie salad dressings contain very little oil but often contain saccharin, which you may want to consider. Most are free when used in moderation.

Product Name	Serving Size	Calories	Exchanges

CONDIMENTS

Product Name	Serving Size	Calories	Exchanges
Bacon bits, *Oscar Mayer*	1 tsp.	7	free in moderation
Bacon crumbles, *Libby's*	1 tsp.	8	free in moderation
Bacon-flavored bits,			
Bac-O's	1 tsp.	13	free in moderation
Durkee	1 tsp.	8	free in moderation
French's	1 tsp.	6	free in moderation
McCormick	1 tsp	9	free in moderation
Barbecue sauce,			
Chris & Pitt's	1 tbsp.	15	free in moderation
Featherweight	1 tbsp.	8	free in moderation
French's Cattlemen's	2 tsp.	17	free in moderation
Heinz, **all flavors**	1 tbsp.	20	free in moderation
Burger sauce, *Hellmann's Big H*	2 tsp.	50	1 F
Catsup,			
Del Monte	1 tbsp.	15	free in moderation
Dia-Mel	1 tbsp.	6	free in moderation
Heinz	1 tbsp.	18	free in moderation
Smucker's	2 tsp.	14	free in moderation
Hot, *Heinz*	1 tbsp.	18	free in moderation
Imitation, *Featherweight*	1 tbsp	6	free in moderation
Chile salsa, green,			
Ortega	2 tbsp.	6	free in moderation
Mild, *Del Monte*	2 tbsp.	10	free in moderation
Chili sauce,			
Del Monte	1 tbsp.	18	free in moderation
Featherweight	1 tbsp.	8	free in moderation
Famous sauce, *Durkee*	1 tbsp	69	1½ F
Hot sauce, *Frank's*	1 tsp.	1	free
Mustard,			
French's, **all flavors**	1 tbsp.	15	free in moderation
Grey Poupon	1 tbsp.	18	free in moderation
Mr. Mustard	1 tsp.	11	free in moderation
Unsalted, *Featherweight*	1 tsp.	5	free in moderation
Peppers,			

Product Name	Serving Size	Calories	Exchanges
Chile,			
Ortega	1 oz.	6	free in moderation
Green, *Del Monte*	1 oz.	5	free in moderation
Green, *Old El Paso*	1 oz.	7	free in moderation
Jalapeño, *Ortega*	1 oz.	7	free in moderation
Hot, *Ortega*	1 oz.	8	free in moderation
Pickles,			
Cauliflower, hot, *Vlasic*	1 oz.	20	1 V
Dill,			
Hamburger chip, *Vlasic*	1 oz.	2	free in moderation
Kosher, *Featherweight*	1 oz.	4	free in moderation
Kosher, *Vlasic*	1 oz.	4	free in moderation
Kosher spears, *Vlasic*	2 spears	4	free in moderation
Whole, *Featherweight*	1 pickle	4	free in moderation
Sliced cucumber, *Featherweight*	1 pickle	12	free in moderation
Relish,			
Dill, *Vlasic*	1 tsp.	1	free
Hamburger, *Heinz*	1 tbsp.	30	1 V
Hot dog, *Heinz*	1 tbsp.	35	1 V
India, *Heinz*	1 tbsp.	35	1 V
Picalilli, *Heinz*	1 tbsp.	30	1 V
Salsa picante,			
Del Monte	1 tbsp	5	free in moderation
Hot & chunky, *Del Monte*	1 tbsp.	4	free in moderation
Salsa roja, mild, *Del Monte*	1 tbsp.	5	free in moderation
Sauce Diable, *Escoffier*	1 tsp.	7	free in moderation
Sauce Robert, *Escoffier*	1 tsp.	7	free in moderation
Seafood cocktail sauce, *Del Monte*	1 tbsp.	18	free in moderation
Steak sauce,			
A-1	1 tbsp.	12	free in moderation
Heinz 57	1 tbsp.	12	free in moderation
Steak Supreme	1 tsp.	7	free in moderation
Taco sauce,			
Ortega	1 tsp.	7	free in moderation
Hot,			
Del Monte	1 tbsp.	4	free in moderation
Old El Paso	1 tbsp.	5	free in moderation
Mild,			
Del Monte	1 tbsp.	4	free in moderation
Old El Paso	1 tbsp.	5	free in moderation
Tartar sauce, *Hellmann's*	2 tsp.	50	1 F

Product Name	Serving Size	Calories	Exchanges
Vinegar, wine, *Regina*	1 oz.	4	free
Worcestershire sauce,			
French's	1 tbsp.	10	free in moderation
Heinz	1 tbsp.	10	free in moderation

GRAVIES

■ Mixes

Au Jus,

Durkee	½ cup prepared	15	free in moderation
French's	¼ cup prepared	8	free in moderation

Brown,

Durkee	¼ cup prepared	15	free in moderation
Durkee Weight Watcher	¼ cup prepared	8	free in moderation
French's	¼ cup prepared	20	½ B
McCormick	¼ cup prepared	91	1 B, ½ F
Pillsbury	½ cup prepared	50	½ B
Spatini Family Style	¼ cup prepared	16	free in moderation
Weight Watchers	¼ cup prepared	6	free in moderation

with Mushrooms,

Durkee	¼ cup prepared	14	free in moderation
Durkee Weight Watcher	¼ cup prepared	12	free in moderation
Weight Watchers	¼ cup prepared	8	free in moderation

with Onions,

Durkee	¼ cup prepared	16	free in moderation
Durkee Weight Watcher	¼ cup prepared	13	free in moderation
Weight Watchers	¼ cup prepared	8	free in moderation

Chicken,

Durkee	¼ cup prepared	22	½ B
Durkee Weight Watcher	¼ cup prepared	10	free in moderation
French's	¼ cup prepared	25	½ B
McCormick	¼ pkg.	85	1 B, ½ F
Pillsbury	½ cup prepared	50	½ B
Weight Watchers	¼ cup prepared	10	free in moderation
Creamy, *Durkee*	¼ cup prepared	39	½ F

Cooking sauce, *Durkee Simmer Sauce,*

Beef	¼ pkg.	42	½ B
Homestyle	¼ pkg.	33	½ B
Italian	¼ pkg.	36	½ B
Flavoring, *Kitchen Bouquet*	1 tsp.	11	free in moderation

Product Name	Serving Size	Calories	Exchanges

Homestyle,

Durkee	¼ cup prepared	18	free in moderation
French's	¼ cup prepared	25	½ B
Pillsbury	½ cup prepared	50	½ B

Mushroom,

Durkee	¼ cup prepared	15	free in moderation
French's	2 tbsp.	10	free in moderation

Onion,

Durkee	2 tbsp.	10	free in moderation
French's	¼ cup prepared	25	½ B
McCormick	¼ pkg.	75	½ B, ½ F

Pork,

Durkee	¼ cup prepared	18	free in moderation
French's	2 tbsp.	10	free in moderation

Swiss steak, *Durkee* .... ¼ cup prepared .... 11 ...... free in moderation

Turkey,

Durkee	2 tbsp.	11	free in moderation
French's	¼ cup prepared	25	½ B

■Canned

Au Jus, *Franco-American*	¼ cup	10	free in moderation
Beef, *Franco-American*	¼ cup	25	½ F
Brown with onions, *Franco-American*	½ cup	25	½ F
Chicken, *Franco-American*	¼ cup	50	1 F
Chicken giblet, *Franco-American*	¼ cup	30	½ F
Mushroom, *Franco-American*	¼ cup	25	½ F
Turkey, *Franco-American*	¼ cup	30	½ F

MAYONNAISE AND SALAD DRESSING

■Mayonnaise and Mayonnaise-type Salad Dressing

Mayonnaise,

Bama	1 tsp.	33	1 F
Best Foods	1 tsp.	35	1 F
Dia-Mel	1 tsp.	35	1 F
Featherweight Soyamaise	1 tsp.	33	1 F
Hellmann's Real	1 tsp.	35	1 F
Weight Watchers, **reduced calorie**	1 tbsp.	40	1 F

Mayonnaise-type salad dressing,

Bama	1 tbsp.	50	1 F

Product Name	Serving Size	Calories	Exchanges
Dia-Mel Diet Whipped	1 tbsp.	24	½ F
Hellmann's Sandwich Spread	2 tsp.	40	1 F

■ Salad Dressing

All flavors, *Weight Watchers*

Salad Surprise Dry Mix	1 tbsp. prepared	2-14, depending on flavor	free in moderation
Bacon, creamy, *Seven Seas*	1 tbsp.	60	1 F

Blue cheese,

Dia-Mel	1 tbsp.	1	free

Chunky,

Seven Seas	1 tbsp.	70	1½ F
Wish-Bone	1 tbsp.	70	1½ F
Wish-Bone Lite Line	1 tbsp.	40	1 F

Imitation low calorie,

Featherweight	1 tbsp.	4	free in moderation

Mix,

Durkee Weight Watcher	1 tbsp. prepared	10	free in moderation
Hidden Valley Ranch	1 tbsp. prepared	36	½ F
Hidden Valley Ranch Milk Recipe	1 tbsp. prepared	56	1 F

Buttermilk,

Seven Seas	1 tbsp.	80	1½ F
Seven Seas Country Spice	1 tbsp.	80	1½ F

Mix,

Hidden Valley Ranch	1 tbsp. prepared	36	½ F
Hidden Valley Ranch Milk Recipe	1 tbsp. prepared	56	1 F

Caesar,

Seven Seas	1 tbsp.	60	1 F
Seven Seas Viva	1 tbsp.	60	1 F
Wish-Bone	1 tbsp.	80	1½ F
Creamy, *Featherweight*	1 tbsp.	14	½ F
Capri, *Seven Seas*	1 tbsp.	70	1½ F

Cucumber,

Creamy,

Dia-Mel	1 tbsp.	1	free
Featherweight	1 tbsp.	12	½ F
Wish-Bone	1 tbsp.	80	1½ F
Wish-Bone Lite Line	1 tbsp.	40	1 F
and Onion, *Featherweight*	1 tbsp.	4	free in moderation

French,

Seven Seas Family Style	1 tbsp.	60	1 F

Product Name	Serving Size	Calories	Exchanges
Wish-Bone Deluxe	1 tbsp.	60	1 F
Wish-Bone Lite Line	1 tbsp.	30	½ F
Wish-Bone Sweet 'N Spicy	1 tbsp.	60	1 F
Wish-Bone Lite Line Sweet 'N Spicy	1 tbsp.	30	½ F
Creamy, *Seven Seas*	1 tbsp.	60	1 F
Garlic, *Wish-Bone*	1 tbsp.	60	1 F
Imitation low calorie, *Featherweight*	1 tbsp.	6	free in moderation
Low sodium, *Featherweight*	1 tbsp.	60	1 F
Mix, *Durkee Weight Watcher*	1 tbsp. prepared	4	free in moderation
Garlic,			
Caesar, *Estee*	1 tbsp.	4	free in moderation
Creamy, *Wish-Bone*	1 tbsp.	80	1½ F
Green Goddess,			
Seven Seas	1 tbsp.	60	1 F
Wish-Bone	1 tbsp.	70	1½ F
Mix, *Hidden Valley Ranch*	1 tbsp. prepared	36	½ F
Herb,			
Estee Herb Garden	1 tbsp.	4	free in moderation
Mix, *Hidden Valley Milk Recipe*	1 tbsp. prepared	56	1 F
and Spices, *Seven Seas*	1 tbsp.	60	1 F
Italian,			
Estee Spicy	1 tbsp.	4	free in moderation
Featherweight	1 tbsp.	4	free in moderation
Seven Seas Family Style	1 tbsp.	70	1½ F
Seven Seas Viva	1 tbsp.	70	1½ F
Wish-Bone	1 tbsp.	80	1½ F
Wish-Bone Lite Line	1 tbsp.	30	½ F
Wish-Bone Robusto	1 tbsp.	80	1½ F
Creamy,			
Seven Seas	1 tbsp.	70	1½ F
Weight Watchers	1 tbsp.	50	1 F
Wish-Bone	1 tbsp.	80	1½ F
Wish-Bone Lite Line	1 tbsp.	30	½ F
Mix, *Durkee Weight Watcher*	1 tbsp. prepared	4	free in moderation
Mix, *Hidden Valley Ranch*	1 tbsp. prepared	36	½ F
Mix, *Hidden Valley Milk Recipe*	1 tbsp. prepared	56	1 F
Mix,			
Durkee Weight Watcher	1 tbsp. prepared	2	free in moderation
Good Seasons, **low-calorie**	1 tbsp. prepared	8	free in moderation

Product Name	Serving Size	Calories	Exchanges

Onion,
  and Chive,

Seven Seas	1 tbsp.	60	1 F
Wish-Bone Lite Line	1 tbsp.	40	1 F
and Cucumber, *Estee*	1 tbsp.	6	free in moderation
Mix, *Hidden Valley Milk Recipe*	1 tbsp. prepared	56	1 F

Red wine vinegar and oil,

Seven Seas	1 tbsp.	60	1 F

Russian,

Weight Watchers	1 tbsp.	50	1 F
Wish-Bone	1 tbsp.	50	1 F
Wish-Bone Lite Line	1 tbsp.	25	½ F
Creamy,			
Seven Seas	1 tbsp.	80	1½ F
Low calorie, *Featherweight*	1 tbsp.	6	free in moderation
Mix, *Durkee Weight Watcher*	1 tbsp. prepared	4	free in moderation

Tahiti, *Dia-Mel*	1 tbsp.	1	free

Thousand Island,

Dia-Mel	1 tbsp.	2	free
Seven Seas	1 tbsp.	50	1 F
Wish-Bone	1 tbsp.	70	1½ F
Wish-Bone Lite Line	1 tbsp.	25	½ F
Mix,			
Durkee Weight Watcher	1 tbsp. prepared	12	free in moderation
Hidden Valley Ranch	1 tbsp. prepared	36	½ F
Yogurt buttermilk, *Estee*	1 tbsp.	1	free

SAUCES

■ Mixes

À la king, *Durkee*	¼ cup prepared	33	½ F
Cheese,			
Durkee	¼ cup prepared	84	1 F, ½ Mk
French's	¼ cup prepared	80	1 F, ½ Mk
Enchilada, *Durkee*	½ cup prepared	28	1 V
Hollandaise,			
Durkee	¼ cup prepared	70	1½ F
French's	3 tbsp. prepared	45	1 F
Lemon butter,			
Durkee Weight Watcher	1 tbsp. prepared	8	free in moderation
Weight Watchers	1 tbsp. prepared	10	free in moderation

Product Name	Serving Size	Calories	Exchanges
Sour cream, *French's*	2½ tbsp. prepared	60	1½ F
Spaghetti,			
Durkee	½ cup prepared	45	½ B, ½ V
French's,			
Italian Style	5 oz. prepared	100	½ B, 1 V, 1 F
Thick Homemade Style	7 oz. prepared	170	1 B, 1 V, 1½ F
McCormick	⅕ pkg.	61	½ B, 1 V
Spatini	1 oz. prepared	20	½ V
with Mushrooms,			
Durkee	½ cup prepared	41	½ B, ½ V
French's	5 oz. prepared	100	½ B, 1 V, 1 F
Stroganoff, *French's*	⅓ cup	100	½ B, 1 F, ½ Mk
Teriyaki, *French's*	2 tbsp.	35	½ B
Tomato, savory, *Durkee*	¼ pkg. prepared	28	1 V
White, *Durkee*	¼ cup prepared	79	1 F, ½ Mk

■ Prepared (in cans or jars)

Product Name	Serving Size	Calories	Exchanges
Cooking sauce,			
Chinese style, *La Sauce* for Chicken	4 oz.	110	1½ B
Enchilada, *Del Monte,* Hot or Mild	½ cup	45	½ B
Italian Style, *La Sauce* for Chicken	3¾ oz.	60	1 B
Mild Mexican, *La Sauce* for Chicken	4½ oz.	70	1 B
Italian, *Contadina*	4 oz.	71	½ B, ½ V, ½ F
Pizza topping,			
Appian Way	6 oz.	100	½ B, 1 V, 1 F
Contadina	½ cup	80	½ B, ½ V, ½ F
Ragú Pizza Quick,			
All flavors	3 tbsp.	35	½ B
Chunky, all flavors	3 tbsp.	45	½ B
with Cheese, *Contadina*	½ cup	90	½ B, ½ V, 1 F
with Pepperoni, *Contadina*	½ cup	80	½ B, ½ V, ½ F
Salsa mexicana, *Contadina*	4 oz.	38	1 V
Spaghetti sauce,			
Featherweight	⅔ cup	80	½ B, ½ V, ½ F
Prego	2 oz.	80	½ B, 1 V, ½ F
Ragú,	4 oz.	80	½ B, ½ V, ½ F
Extra Thick and Zesty	4 oz.	100	½ B, 1 V, 1 F
Homestyle	4 oz.	70	½ B, ½ V, ½ F

Product Name	Serving Size	Calories	Exchanges
Flavored with meat,			
Prego	2 oz.	80	½ B, 1 V, ½ F
Ragú	4 oz.	80	½ B, ½ V, ½ F
Ragú Extra Thick and Zesty	4 oz.	100	½ B, 1 V, 1 F
Ragú Homestyle	4 oz.	80	½ B, ½ V, ½ F
Marinara, *Ragú*	4 oz.	90	½ B, ½ V, 1 F
with Mushrooms,			
Prego	2 oz.	70	½ B, 1 V, ½ F
Ragú	4 oz.	90	½ B, ½ V, 1 F
Ragú Extra Thick and Zesty	4 oz.	110	½ B, 1 V, 1 F
Ragú Homestyle	4 oz.	70	½ B, ½ V, ½ F

SEASONINGS

Product Name	Serving Size	Calories	Exchanges
Flavoring extracts (almond, anise, banana, lemon, maple, orange, peppermint, vanilla, etc., all brands)	1 tsp.	4-15	free
Seasoning mixes,			
Season-All	1 tsp.	4	free in moderation
Salad Supreme	1 tsp.	11	free in moderation
Beef stew, *French's*	⅙ pkg.	25	½ B
Burger,			
Makes a Better Burger	⅓ oz. dry	30	½ B
with Onions, *Makes a Better Burger*	⅓ oz. dry	30	½ B
Chili,			
French's Chili-O	⅙ pkg.	25	½ B
McCormick	⅙ pkg.	50	½ B
Enchilada, *French's*	¼ pkg.	30	½ B
Ground beef with onions, *French's*	¼ pkg.	25	½ B
Hamburger, *French's*	¼ pkg.	25	½ B
Meat marinade,			
Durkee	⅛ cup prepared	12	free in moderation
French's	⅛ pkg	10	free in moderation
Meatball, *French's*	¼ pkg.	35	½ B
Meatloaf,			
Contadina	1 tbsp.	35	½ B
French's	⅛ pkg.	20	½ B
Sloppy Joe,			
French's	⅛ pkg.	16	free in moderation
McCormick	⅙ pkg.	45	½ B

Product Name	Serving Size	Calories	Exchanges
Taco, *French's*	⅙ pkg.	20	½ B
Spices (allspice, basil, cinnamon, cloves, garlic powder, ginger, nutmeg paprika, parsley, pepper, sage, tarragon, thyme, etc., all brands)	1 tsp.	3-15	free
Wine, cooking, *Regina*	¼ cup	2	free in moderation

8

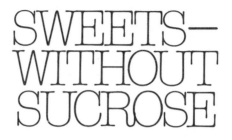

SWEETS—
WITHOUT
SUCROSE

☐ Beverages
☐ Candy and gum
☐ Cookies and bars
☐ Desserts
☐ Jams, jellies, and preserves
☐ Table-top sugar substitutes
☐ Toppings and syrups

These products—sweetened with aspartame (NutraSweet), fructose, saccharin, and sorbitol—can help satisfy your sweet tooth without upsetting your blood sugar levels. Foods made with sugar substitutes offer diabetics the sweet taste of sucrose (table sugar) without some of its disadvantages. Recent research suggests that moderate amounts of sucrose taken with a balanced meal may not cause the rapid rise in blood sugar that was formerly feared, but this doesn't mean that you can freely consume sugar-sweetened foods. In particular, you should not eat them between meals unless you're an insulin-dependent diabetic performing vigorous physical exercise. Even when consumed in moderation and with meals, sugar provides a substantial number of "empty" calories. Choosing a sugary food such as a cookie over a bread exchange such as potatoes or a whole-wheat roll means losing important minerals, vitamins, and fiber.

The American Diabetes Association recommends that diabetics restrict sugar consumption.* Be aware that sugar masquerades under many names on food labels: dextrose, glucose, sucrose (all the "—ose" names), corn syrup, corn syrup solids, sorghum, sugar cane syrup, brown sugar, honey, maple syrup, and molasses. All are sugar, and you should avoid them unless your physician tells you otherwise.

Many "dietetic," "artificially sweetened," "non-sugar-sweetened," and "reduced-calorie" products are of some value as alternatives to the diabetic consumer. But you should consider these points:

•A "dietetic" food is not necessarily a "diabetic" food. "Dietetic" can also refer to low sodium or reduced fat.

•While some dietetic cookies and candies offer a reduced sugar and carbohydrate content because they're sweetened with one of the products discussed below, they may contain *more* fat and calories than their sugar-sweetened counterparts—a point to consider if you're trying to lose weight.

•Many non-sugar-sweetened products are quite expensive, yet provide few nutritional benefits.

•The only completely nonnutritive (calorie-free) sweetener available in the U.S. today is saccharin, which has been shown to cause cancer in laboratory animals.

The following sugar substitutes are most commonly found in brand-name products:

Aspartame (**NutraSweet**) is a low-calorie sweetener synthesized from two amino acids, aspartic acid and phenylalanine. Although it is caloric (4 calories per gram), it is almost 200 times as sweet as sucrose and can thus be used in very small amounts—one-tenth of a calorie replaces a teaspoon of sugar (16 calories). Since 1981, the FDA has approved its use in cold cereals, drink mixes, sugarless gums, gelatins, puddings, dairy products, toppings, and as a table-top sweetener (**Equal**). In July 1983, it was also approved for use in diet soft drinks. Most bottlers use some saccharin along with the aspartame. Check the label to be sure.

Aspartame is metabolized as a protein, and thus has no effect on blood sugar levels. It has no aftertaste, and no serious side effects have been identified to date. However, aspartame decomposes to yield small amounts of methanol, which some scientists feel may be harmful.

Fructose, a common monosaccharide (simple sugar), occurs naturally in sweet fruits and berries. It contains 4 calories per gram (the same as sucrose), but is one-and-a-half to two times as sweet as sucrose, depending on the temperature at which it is served. Absorbed more slowly and metabolized differently than sucrose, fructose causes a smaller increase in blood sugar levels. However, it is not recommended for untreated or poorly controlled diabetics, and its caloric content must be included in your meal plan.

Saccharin, the only artificial, nonnutritive sweetener in use in the U.S. since cyclamates were banned in 1969, contains no calories and is 300 to 500 times as sweet as sucrose. However, saccharin has been shown to cause cancer in laboratory animals, and its use may increase the risk of certain kinds of cancer in humans. The FDA proposed a partial ban of saccharin in 1977, but public protest was so strong that Congress imposed a moratorium on the ban extending through August 1983. Recently, this moratorium was extended again

---

* *Diabetes Care* 2(6):520,1979

through April 1985.

Many people find saccharin has a bitter aftertaste. Saccharin has no effect on blood sugar levels, but in light of its potential hazards, it should be used in moderation. All products containing saccharin are required to display a warning label.

Sorbitol, like fructose, is a nutritive sugar substitute, technically called a sugar alcohol. It also contains 4 calories per gram and is about half as sweet as sucrose. Found in many "sugar-free" candies and desserts, it is absorbed more slowly than sucrose and metabolized differently. Sorbitol does not cause large rises in blood sugar levels in well-controlled diabetics, but it has been shown to cause diarrhea when used in large amounts (more than 30 to 50 grams per day). A typical hard candy contains about 2 grams of sorbitol.

In this chapter we identify the type of sugar substitute used in each product, as well as the calories and exchanges. Be aware that many of the table-top sugar substitutes contain one of the sweeteners listed above in combination with such ingredients as dextrin (a polysaccharide, or complex sugar, composed of a chain of glucose molecules); dextrose (the commercial name for glucose produced from cornstarch); and lactose (a disaccharide, or double sugar, composed of glucose and galactose). All products containing these substances have a small number of calories, and, when used in large quantities, may affect your blood sugar level.

The table below will help you compare nutritive (caloric) and nonnutritive (calorie-free) sweeteners at a glance.

COMMON SWEETENERS

Sweetener	Calories per gram	Sweetness relative to sugar	Effect on blood sugar	Advantages	Disadvantages
Sucrose (Table sugar)	4	————	Increases blood sugar levels when eaten alone; effect modified by other foods	Fast-acting and effective for treatment of hypoglycemia	Increases blood sugar levels; promotes tooth decay; provides empty calories
Aspartame (*NutraSweet*)	4	200 times as sweet	None	Very low in calories; no aftertaste	Breaks down at high temperatures and cannot be used in cooking; decomposes slowly in solution; effects of decomposition products still being debated
Fructose	4	1½ to 2 times as sweet	Substantially less increase than sucrose in well-controlled diabetics	Clean taste without aftertaste	Contains the same number of calories per gram as sucrose, although slightly less is needed; long-term effects on diabetics not known

Sweetener	Calories per gram	Sweetness relative to sugar	Effect on blood sugar	Advantages	Disadvantages
Saccharin	0	300 to 500 times as sweet	None	No calories; widely available	Causes cancer in laboratory animals and may increase risk in humans; may be withdrawn from market; bitter aftertaste
Sorbitol	4	Half as sweet	Gradual, moderate increase in well-controlled diabetics	Cool, sweet taste; slow absorption	Contains the same number of calories per gram as sucrose, but more is needed; causes diarrhea in large amounts; long-term effects on diabetics not known

Product Name	Serving Size	Sweetener	Calories	Exchanges

BEVERAGES

■ Carbonated

Product Name	Serving Size	Sweetener	Calories	Exchanges
Canada Dry Ginger Ale, sugar-free	8 fl. oz.	saccharin	2	free
Coke, Diet,	6 fl. oz.	saccharin	0.5	free
Caffeine-free	6 fl. oz.	saccharin	0.5	free
Diet Rite Cola, sugar-free	6 fl. oz.	saccharin	0	free
Fresca	6 fl. oz.	saccharin	1.8	free
Dr Pepper, sugar-free,	6 fl. oz.	saccharin	1.5	free
Caffeine-free (*Pepper Free*)	6 fl. oz.	saccharin	1.5	free
Mr. Pibb, sugar-free	6 fl. oz.	saccharin	0.6	free
Pepsi, diet,	6 fl. oz.	saccharin	0.5	free
Caffeine-free (*Pepsi Free*)	6 fl. oz.	saccharin	0.5	free
Pepsi Light	6 fl. oz.	saccharin	0.5	free
Ramblin' Root Beer, sugar-free	6 fl. oz.	saccharin	0.7	free
RC 100, sugar-free, caffeine-free	6 fl. oz.	saccharin	0	free
Sprite, sugar-free	6 fl. oz.	saccharin	1.4	free
Tab	6 fl. oz.	saccharin	0.5	free
Caffeine-free	6 fl. oz.	saccharin	0.3	free

■ Mixes

Product Name	Serving Size	Sweetener	Calories	Exchanges
All flavors, *Wyler's Sugar Free*	8 fl. oz.	aspartame*	4	free

*Aspartame is the generic name for *NutraSweet.*

Product Name	Serving Size	Sweetener	Calories	Exchanges
Cherry,				
Calorie Control	8 fl. oz.	aspartame*	6	free
Kool-Aid Sugar Free	8 fl. oz.	aspartame*	4	free
Cocoa, hot,				
Alba, **all flavors**	1 env.	aspartame*	60	1 Mk
Calorie Control	6 fl. oz.	aspartame*	40	½ Mk
Superman	1 env.	aspartame*	70	1 Mk
Grape, *Kool-Aid Sugar Free*	8 fl. oz.	aspartame*	4	free
Iced tea, lemon-flavored, sugar-free, *Lipton*	8 fl. oz.	aspartame*	4	free
Lemonade,				
Kool-Aid Sugar Free	8 fl. oz.	aspartame*	4	free
Pink, *Calorie Control*	8 fl. oz.	aspartame*	6	free
Milkshakes, chocolate or vanilla,				
Alba 77 Fit 'N Frosty	1 env.	aspartame*	70	1 Mk
Calorie Control	12 fl. oz.	aspartame*	70	1 Mk
Orange, *Calorie Control*	8 fl. oz.	aspartame*	6	free
Punch,				
Sunshine, *Kool-Aid Sugar Free*	8 fl. oz.	aspartame*	4	free
Tropical fruit,				
Calorie Control	8 fl. oz.	aspartame*	6	free
Kool-Aid Sugar Free	8 fl. oz.	aspartame*	4	free

CANDY AND GUM

Product Name	Serving Size	Sweetener	Calories	Exchanges
Chocolate bars,				
Almond, *Estee*	2 squares	sorbitol	60	½ B, ½ F
Bittersweet, *Estee*	2 squares	sorbitol	60	½ B, ½ F
Coconut, *Estee*	2 squares	sorbitol	60	½ B, ½ F
Crunch, *Estee*	2 squares	sorbitol	45	½ B, ½ F
Fruit and nut, *Estee*	2 squares	sorbitol	60	½ B, ½ F
Milk, *Estee*	2 squares	sorbitol	60	½ B, ½ F
Toasted bran, *Estee*	2 squares	sorbitol	60	½ B, ½ F
Chocolate-coated raisins, *Estee*	10 candies	sorbitol	50	½ B, ½ F
Estee-ets	8 candies	sorbitol	56	½ B, ½ F
Gum,				
Chewels	1 piece	sorbitol/ mannitol	8	free in moderation
Orbit	1 piece	sorbitol	8	free in moderation

---

*Aspartame is the generic name for *NutraSweet*.

Product Name	Serving Size	Sweetener	Calories	Exchanges
Trident,	1 piece	sorbitol	5	free in moderation
Bubble gum	1 piece	sorbitol	7	free in moderation
Gum drops, *Estee*	7 drops	sorbitol/ fructose	21	½ Fr
Hard candies,				
Eda's Sugar Free	1 candy	sorbitol	9	free in moderation
Estee	2 candies	sorbitol	25	½ Fr
Sorbee, **all flavors**	1 candy	sorbitol	9	free in moderation
Lollipops, *Estee*	1 lollipop	sorbitol	12	free in moderation
Mints,				
Certs Sugar Free	1 piece	sorbitol	6	free in moderation
Estee	5 mints	sorbitol	20	1 Fr
Trident, **round**	1 piece	sorbitol	8	free in moderation
Trident, **square**	1 piece	sorbitol	10	free in moderation
Ultamints	10 candies	sorbitol	10	free in moderation
Velamints	1 candy	sorbitol	9	free in moderation
Peanut butter cups, *Estee*	2 candies	sorbitol	90	½ B, 1 F
T.V. mix, *Estee*	10 candies	sorbitol	88	½ B, 1 F

COOKIES AND BARS

Product Name	Serving Size	Sweetener	Calories	Exchanges
Chocolate,				
Featherweight	1 cookie	sorbitol	28	½ B
Chip,				
Estee	2 cookies	fructose	50	½ B, ½ F
Featherweight	1 cookie	sorbitol	40	½ B
Coated wafers, *Estee*	1 wafer	sorbitol	120	1 B, 1 F
Creme-filled wafers, *Estee*	3 wafers	sorbitol	60	½ B, ½ F
Snack wafers, *Estee*	1 wafer	sorbitol	80	½ B, 1 F
Wafers, *Featherweight*	1 wafer	sorbitol	30	½ B
Coconut fudge, *Estee*	2 cookies	fructose	50	½ B, ½ F
Estee **Duplex Sandwich**	1 cookie	sorbitol	60	½ B, ½ F
Lemon,				
Featherweight	1 cookie	sorbitol	40	½ F
Sandwich, *Estee*	1 cookie	sorbitol	50	½ B, ½ F
Thins, *Estee*	2 cookies	fructose	50	½ B, ½ F
Oatmeal raisin, *Estee*	2 cookies	fructose	50	½ B, ½ F
Peanut butter creme wafers, *Featherweight*	1 wafer	sorbitol	40	½ B
Strawberry snack wafers, *Estee*	1 wafer	sorbitol	80	½ B, 1 F

Product Name	Serving Size	Sweetener	Calories	Exchanges
Vanilla,				
Featherweight	1 cookie	sorbitol	40	½ B
Creme-filled wafers, *Estee*	3 wafers	sorbitol	60	½ B, ½ F
Creme wafers, *Featherweight*	1 wafer	sorbitol	40	½ B
Snack wafers, *Estee*	1 wafer	sorbitol	80	½ B, 1 F
Thins, *Estee*	2 cookies	fructose	50	½ B, ½ F

DESSERTS

Product Name	Serving Size	Sweetener	Calories	Exchanges
Cake,				
Apple raisin spice, *Weight Watchers*	2.6 oz.	fructose	160	1 B, 1 F, 1 Fr
Carrot, *Weight Watchers*	2.6 oz.	fructose	150	1 B, 1 F, 1 Fr
Mix,				
Chocolate, *Dia-Mel*	⅒ cake	sorbitol	100	1 B, 1 F
Chocolate, *Estee*	⅒ cake	fructose	90	1 B, ½ Fr
Lemon, *Dia-Mel*	⅒ cake	sorbitol	100	1 B, 1 F
Lemon, *Estee*	⅒ cake	fructose	80	1 B, ½ Fr
Pound, *Dia-Mel*	⅒ cake	sorbitol	100	1 B, 1 F
Spice, *Dia-Mel*	⅒ cake	sorbitol	100	1 B, 1 F
White, *Estee*	⅒ cake	fructose	80	1 B, ½ Fr
Cobbler,				
Apple, *Weight Watchers*	4½ oz.	fructose	150	1 B, ½ F, 1½ Fr
Black cherry, *Weight Watchers*	4½ oz.	fructose	150	1 B, ½ F, 1½ Fr
Gel,				
All flavors, *Estee*	½ cup	fructose	40	1 Fr
Ready-to-eat, strawberry, *Estee*	4 oz.	fructose	40	1 Fr
Gelatin,				
All flavors,				
Calorie Control	3 fl. oz.	aspartame*	6	free in moderation
Dia-Mel	½ cup	aspartame*	8	free in moderation
D-Zerta	½ cup	saccharin	8	free in moderation
Featherweight	½ cup	aspartame*	10	free in moderation
Featherweight	½ cup	saccharin	10	free in moderation
Ready-to-eat, *Dia-Mel* *Gel-A-Thin*	4 oz.	saccharin	2	free
Pudding,				
All flavors, *Featherweight*	½ cup	aspartame*	12	½ Fr
Butterscotch,				
Dia-Mel	½ cup	aspartame*	50	½ Mk
D-Zerta	½ cup	saccharin	70	½ B, ½ Mk

*Aspartame is the generic name for *NutraSweet*.

Product Name	Serving Size	Sweetener	Calories	Exchanges
Featherweight	4 oz.	saccharin	50	1 B
Chocolate,				
Dia-Mel	½ cup	aspartame*	50	½ Mk
D-Zerta	½ cup	saccharin	70	½ B, ½ Mk
Estee	½ cup	fructose	90	1 Fr, ½ Mk
Featherweight	4 oz.	saccharin	60	1 B
Instant, all flavors,				
Calorie Control	3 fl. oz.	aspartame*	50	½ Mk
Lemon, *Estee*	½ cup	fructose	100	1 B, 1 Fr
Vanilla,				
Dia-Mel	½ cup	aspartame*	50	½ Mk
D-Zerta	½ cup	saccharin	70	½ B, ½ Mk
Estee	½ cup	fructose	85	1 Fr, ½ Mk
Featherweight	4 oz.	saccharin	50	1 B

JAMS, JELLIES, AND PRESERVES

Product Name	Serving Size	Sweetener	Calories	Exchanges
All flavors, *Dia-Mel*	1 tsp.	saccharin	2	free
Apple,				
Jelly, imitation,				
Featherweight **low-calorie**	1 tbsp.	saccharin	6	free in moderation
Featherweight **reduced-calorie**	1 tbsp.	fructose	16	½ Fr
Smucker's Slenderella	2 tsp.	———[1]	16	½ Fr
Apricot,				
Jam, imitation,				
Smucker's Slenderella	2 tsp.	———[1]	16	½ Fr
Low-sugar spread, *Smucker's*	2 tsp.	———[1]	16	½ Fr
Preserves, imitation, *Featherweight* **calorie-reduced**	1 tbsp.	fructose	16	½ Fr
and Pineapple preserves, imitation, *Featherweight* **low-calorie**	1 tbsp.	saccharin	6	free in moderation
Blackberry,				
Jelly, imitation,				
Featherweight **calorie-reduced**	1 tbsp.	fructose	16	½ Fr
Smucker's Single Service	1 pkg. (⅜ oz.)	saccharin	4	free
Smucker's Slenderella	2 tsp.	———[1]	16	½ Fr
Low-Sugar Spread, *Smucker's*	2 tsp.	———[1]	16	½ Fr
Preserves, imitation, *Featherweight* **calorie-reduced**	1 tbsp.	fructose	16	½ Fr

---

*Aspartame is the generic name for NutraSweet.
[1]Made with half the sugar of regular product. No other sweeteners used.

Product Name	Serving Size	Sweetener	Calories	Exchanges
Boysenberry,				
Jam, imitation,				
Smucker's Slenderella	2 tsp.	———[1]	16	½ Fr
Low-Sugar Spread, *Smucker's*	2 tsp.	———[1]	16	½ Fr
Cherry,				
Jelly, imitation,				
Featherweight **calorie-reduced**	1 tbsp.	fructose	16	½ Fr
Featherweight **low-calorie**	1 tbsp.	saccharin	6	free in moderation
Smucker's Single Service	1 pkg. (⅜ oz.)	saccharin	4	free
Smucker's Slenderella	2 tsp.	———[1]	16	½ Fr
Low-sugar Spread, *Smucker's*	2 tsp.	———[1]	16	½ Fr
Grape,				
Jelly, imitation,				
Featherweight **calorie-reduced**	1 tbsp.	fructose	16	½ Fr
Featherweight **low-calorie**	1 tbsp.	saccharin	6	free in moderation
Smucker's	2 tsp.	saccharin	2	free
Smucker's Single Service	1 pkg. (⅜ oz.)	saccharin	4	free
Smucker's Slenderella	2 tsp.	———[1]	16	½ Fr
Lite Spread, *Welch's*	2 tsp.	———[2]	20	½ Fr
Low-Sugar Spread, *Smucker's*	2 tsp.	———[1]	16	½ Fr
Orange marmalade,				
Imitation,				
Featherweight **calorie-reduced**	1 tbsp.	fructose	16	½ Fr
Smucker's Slenderella	2 tsp.	———[1]	16	½ Fr
Low-sugar Spread, *Smucker's*	2 tsp.	———[1]	16	½ Fr
Peach preserves, imitation,				
Featherweight **calorie-reduced**	1 tbsp.	fructose	16	½ Fr
Featherweight **low-calorie**	1 tbsp.	saccharin	6	free in moderation
Plum jelly, *Featherweight* **calorie-reduced**	1 tbsp.	fructose	16	½ Fr
Raspberry preserves, imitation, *Featherweight* **calorie-reduced**	1 tbsp.	fructose	16	½ Fr
Red raspberry low-sugar spread, *Smucker's*	2 tsp.	———[1]	16	½ Fr
Strawberry,				
Jam, imitation,				
Smucker's	2 tsp.	saccharin	2	free
Smucker's Slenderella	2 tsp.	———[1]	16	½ Fr
Jelly, *Featherweight* **calorie-reduced**	1 tbsp.	fructose	16	½ Fr
Lite spread, *Welch's*	2 tsp.	———[2]	20	½ Fr

[1]Made with half the sugar of regular product. No other sweetener used.
[2]Made with one-third less sugar than regular product. No other sweetener used.

Product Name	Serving Size	Sweetener	Calories	Exchanges
Low-sugar spread, *Smucker's*	2 tsp.	———[1]	16	½ Fr
Preserves, imitation,				
Featherweight calorie-reduced	1 tbsp.	fructose	16	½ Fr
Featherweight low-calorie	1 tbsp.	saccharin	6	free in moderation

TABLE-TOP SUGAR SUBSTITUTES

Product Name	Serving Size	Sweetener	Calories	Exchanges
Calorie-free sweetening, *Featherweight*	3 drops	saccharin	0	free
Equal	1 packet	aspartame*	4	free
Equal Sweet-tabs	1 tablet	aspartame*	0	free
Fructose, *Estee,*				
Bulk or packets	2 tsp.	fructose	24	½ Fr
Liquid	1 tsp.	fructose	20	½ Fr
Saccharin tablets, *Featherweight*	1 tablet	saccharin	0	free
Sprinkle Sweet	1 tsp.	saccharin	2	free
SugarTwin,				
Bulk brown	1 tsp.	saccharin	2	free
Bulk white	1 tsp.	saccharin	1.5	free
Packets	1 packet	saccharin	3	free
Sweet'ner, Weight Watchers	1 packet	saccharin	3.5	free
Sweet'n-It, Dia-Mel	6 drops	saccharin	0	free
Sweet 'N Low,				
White	1 packet or ⅓ tsp.	saccharin	3.5	free
Brown	⅒ tsp.	saccharin	2	free
Liquid	10 drops	saccharin	0	free
Sweet 10	⅛ tsp.	saccharin	0	free

TOPPINGS AND SYRUPS

Product Name	Serving Size	Sweetener	Calories	Exchanges
Blueberry, *Featherweight* calorie-reduced	1 tbsp.	fructose	14	½ Fr
Chocolate, *Dia-Mel*	1 tbsp.	saccharin	6	free in moderation
Pancake,				
Dia-Mel	1 tbsp.	saccharin	1	free
Featherweight calorie-reduced	1 tbsp.	fructose	12	½ Fr
Whipped, mix, reduced-calorie, *D-Zerta*	1 tbsp.	saccharin	8	free in moderation

---

*Aspartame is the generic name for *NutraSweet.*
[1]Made with half the sugar of regular product. No other sweeteners used.

9

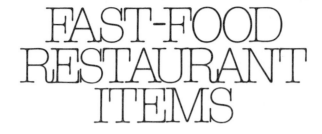

FAST-FOOD RESTAURANT ITEMS

☐ Arby's
☐ Burger King
☐ Dairy Queen/Brazier
☐ Hardee's
☐ Long John Silver's
☐ Kentucky Fried Chicken
☐ McDonald's
☐ Roy Rogers
☐ Taco Bell
☐ Wendy's

Fast-food restaurants, a familiar part of the American landscape, offer convenience, reasonable prices, and—most important for the diabetic—standardized portions. The stringent portion control practiced by most fast-food restaurants means that the exchanges listed here, while based on average portion sizes, will vary little from one outlet to the next. On the other hand, these foods are often loaded with calories, saturated fat, cholesterol, and salt, and deficient in certain vitamins (particularly A) and fiber. That means you should be aware of what you're eating and take steps to make your meal as nutritious as possible.

You *can* work these foods into your meal plan in moderation. With all the specialties (such as burgers, fried chicken, fried fish, pizza, and roast beef sandwiches) and sidelines (such as beverages, desserts, cole slaw, french fries, and onion rings) available, you can afford to be choosy.

Let's look at some typical fast-food items. A "jumbo" burger, for instance, might be composed of a large roll (3 bread exchanges), ground beef (3 meat exchanges and 1½ fat exchanges), pickles, lettuce, and catsup (free exchanges), and mayonnaise or a mayonnaise-based "special sauce" (3 teaspoons equaling 3 fat exchanges), for a total of 570 calories. You could reduce the number of calories and fat exchanges substantially by choosing a regular-sized sandwich, and by asking the counterperson to "hold the mayo" or "hold the sauce." For example, by "holding the mayo" on a Burger King Whopper (630 calories; 3½ bread, 3 meat, and 5 fat exchanges), you'll save 3 fat exchanges (135 calories). Changing your order to a "Whopper Jr., hold the mayo" will give you 320 calories (2 bread, 1½ meat, and 2 fat exchanges), saving you 310 calories. If you're eating a roast beef sandwich (about 350 calories; 2 bread, 2½ meat, and 1½ fat exchanges), why not avoid adding table condiments such as mayonnaise or horseradish sauce (50 calories; 1 fat exchange per tablespoon)? And skip the cole slaw if it seems to have lots of dressing (1 fat exchange per teaspoon).

Many people think they're saving calories by choosing a fish or chicken sandwich over a beef item. Usually, this isn't the case. While the fish and chicken you cook at home *are* lower in fat than beef, these items are served breaded and fried in fast-food restaurants, adding lots of calories. Often, a plain burger is a better

choice. Before you go to a fast-food restaurant, take some time to examine the exchange values for the products offered. If you do choose a fish sandwich (typically composed of fish, breading, fat from frying, a bun, and tartar sauce; about 410 calories; 2½ bread, 1 meat, 3½ fat exchanges), you'll fit it into your meal plan more easily if you ask for no tartar sauce (saving 3 fat exchanges), and perhaps eat only half of the bun (saving 1 bread exchange). Of course, you'll want to avoid entirely items such as shakes, ice cream, pies, cookies, sundaes, and sugar-sweetened soft drinks, because of their high sugar content.

Watching out for nutrition doesn't have to be all avoidance, though. You can take *positive* steps to increase the nutritional value of your fast-food meal. After choosing your main dishes wisely, accompany your meal with a salad of crisp, fresh vegetables from the salad bar found in many fast-food restaurants these days. Add lettuce, tomato (high in vitamin C), and green pepper (high in vitamins C and A) to your burger. Drink juice, skim milk, or ice water with your meal, rather than a soft drink. Choices like these will help make up for *some* of the missing vitamins and fiber, but you should also follow the American Diabetes Association Committee on Food and Nutrition's recommendations and eat a carefully chosen variety of fruit, vegetables, milk products, and whole grains during the rest of the day to help ensure nutritional adequacy.*

It's up to you. If you choose to eat in fast-food restaurants, you can still make the meal as nutritious as possible.

*Diabetes Care 3(2):389, 1980.

Product Name	Serving Size	Calories	Exchanges

ARBY'S

Roast Beef sandwich,

Regular	5 oz.	350	2 B, 2½ M, 1½ F
Deluxe	8¼ oz.	486	3 B, 3 M, 2½ F
Junior	3 oz.	220	1½ B, 1½ M, 1 F
Super	9¾ oz.	620	4 B, 3 M, 4 F
Beef 'N Cheddar sandwich	6 oz.	484	3 B, 3 M, 2½ F
Chicken Breast sandwich	7¼ oz.	585	3½ B, 3 M, 4 F
Ham 'N Cheese sandwich	8¼ oz.	484	3 B, 3 M, 2½ F
Potato cakes (2)	3½ oz.	190	1½ B, 2 F
French fries	2½ oz.	216	1½ B, 2½ F
Arby sauce	1 tbsp.	15	free in moderation
Horsey sauce	1 tbsp.	50	1 F

BURGER KING

Hamburger,	3.9 oz.	290	2 B, 1½ M, 1½ F
with Cheese	4.4 oz.	350	2 B, 2 M, 2 F
Double meat hamburger,	6.0 oz.	430	2 B, 3 M, 2½ F
with Cheese	6.3 oz.	530	2 B, 4 M, 4 F
Whopper,	9.2 oz.	630	3½ B, 3 M, 5 F
with Cheese	10.2 oz.	740	3½ B, 3½ M, 7 F
Double Beef Whopper	11.9 oz.	850	3½ B, 5 M, 7½ F
with Cheese	12.9 oz.	950	3½ B, 6 M, 8½ F
Whopper Jr.,	5.1 oz.	370	2 B, 1½ M, 3½ F
with Cheese	5.6 oz.	420	2 B, 2 M, 4 F
French fries, regular	2.4 oz.	210	1½ B, 2½ F
Onion rings, regular	2.7 oz.	270	2 B, 3 F

DAIRY QUEEN / BRAZIER

Hamburger,

Single,	5.1 oz.	360	2 B, 2 M, 2½ F
with Cheese	5.6 oz.	410	2 B, 3 M, 2½ F
Double,	7.3 oz.	530	2 B, 4½ M, 3 F
with Cheese	8.5 oz.	650	2 B, 5½ M, 4½ F
Triple,	9.6 oz.	710	2 B, 6 M, 5½ F
with Cheese	10.6 oz.	820	2½ B, 7 M, 6 F
Hot dog,	3.5 oz.	280	1½ B, 1 M, 2½ F
with Cheese	4.0 oz.	330	1½ B, 1½ M, 3 F

Product Name	Serving Size	Calories	Exchanges
with Chili	4.5 oz.	320	1½ B, 1½ M, 3 F
Super,	6.2 oz.	520	3 B, 2 M, 4½ F
with Cheese	6.9 oz.	580	3 B, 2 M, 6 F
with Chili	7.7 oz.	570	3 B, 2 M, 5½ F
Chicken sandwich	7.8 oz.	670	3 B, 3 M, 6½ F
Fish sandwich,	6.0 oz.	400	3 B, 2 M, 2 F
with Cheese	6.3 oz.	440	2½ B, 3 M, 2½ F
French fries,			
Regular	2.5 oz.	200	1½ B, 2 F
Large	4.0 oz.	320	2½ B, 3 F
Onion rings	3.0 oz.	280	2 B, 3 F

HARDEE'S

Product Name	Serving Size	Calories	Exchanges
Hamburger	3.9 oz.	305	2 B, 1½ M, 2 F
Cheeseburger,	4.1 oz.	335	2 B, 2 M, 2 F
Bacon	8.6 oz.	686	3 B, 4 M, 6 F
Quarter-pound	6.7 oz.	506	3 B, 3 M, 3 F
Big Deluxe burger	8.8 oz.	546	3 B, 3½ M, 3 F
Hot dog	4.2 oz.	346	2 B, 1 M, 3½ F
Chicken Fillet sandwich	6.8 oz.	510	2½ B, 3 M, 3½ F
Big Fish sandwich	6.9 oz.	514	3½ B, 1½ M, 4½ F
Hot Ham and Cheese sandwich	5.2 oz.	376	2½ B, 2 M, 2 F
Roast Beef sandwich,	5.0 oz.	377	2½ B, 2 M, 2 F
Big	5.9 oz.	418	2 B, 3 M, 2½ F
French fries,			
Small	2.5 oz.	239	1½ B, 3 F
Large	4.0 oz.	381	3 B, 4 F
Biscuit,			
Plain	2.9 oz.	274	2 B, 3 F
Bacon and egg	4.0 oz.	405	2 B, 1½ M, 4 F
with Egg	5.6 oz.	383	2½ B, 1 M, 3½ F
with Ham	3.8 oz.	350	2½ B, 1 M, 3 F
and Egg	6.5 oz.	458	2½ B, 2 M, 4 F
with Sausage	4.0 oz.	413	2½ B, 1 M, 4 F
and Egg	5.7 oz.	521	2½ B, 1½ M, 6 F
with Steak	4.7 oz.	419	2½ B, 1 M, 4 F
and Egg	5.7 oz.	527	2½ B, 2 M, 5½ F
Fried egg, medium	1.8 oz.	108	1 M, 1 F

Product Name	Serving Size	Calories	Exchanges

KENTUCKY FRIED CHICKEN*

Original Recipe,

Drumstick	1.7 oz.	117	½ B, 1½ M
Keel	3.4 oz.	236	½ B, 3 M, 1 F
Side Breast	2.5 oz.	199	½ B, 2 M, 1 F
Thigh	3.1 oz.	257	½ B, 2½ M, 2 F
Wing	1.5 oz.	136	½ B, 1½ M, ½ F

Extra Crispy,

Drumstick	2.1 oz.	155	½ B, 1½ M, 1 F
Keel	3.7 oz.	297	1 B, 3 M, 1½ F
Side Breast	3.0 oz.	286	1 B, 2 M, 2½ F
Thigh	3.8 oz.	343	1 B, 3 M, 2½ F
Wing	1.9 oz.	201	½ B, 1½ M, 2 F
Chicken Breast Filet sandwich	5.6 oz.	436	2 B, 3 M, 3 F
Cole slaw	3.2 oz.	121	½ B, ½ V, 1½ F
Corn on the cob	5½ inches long	169	2 B, ½ F
Gravy	0.5 oz.	23	½ F
Kentucky Fries	3.0 oz.	184	2 B, 1 F
Mashed potatoes	3.0 oz.	63	1 B
Roll	0.7 oz.	64	1 B

LONG JOHN SILVER'S

Breaded Clams	5 oz.	617	4 B, 1½ M, 6 F
Breaded Oysters	6 pieces	441	3½ B, 1 M, 3 F
Chicken Planks	4 pieces	457	2½ B, 3 M, 2½ F
Fish with Batter	2 pieces	366	1½ B, 2½ M, 3 F
Fish with Batter	3 pieces	549	2 B, 4 M, 4 F
Ocean Scallops	6 pieces	283	2 B, 1 M, 2 F
Shrimp with Batter	6 pieces	268	2 B, ½ M, 2½ F
Clam chowder	8 oz.	107	½ B, ½ F, ½ Mk
Cole slaw	4 oz.	138	½ B, 1½ F, 1 V
Corn on the cob	1 ear	176	2 B, 1 F
French Fryes	3 oz.	288	2 B, 3½ F
Hushpuppies	3 pieces	153	1½ B, 1 F

---

*All amounts are edible portion only. Exchanges mathematically calculated from existing caloric information provided by Kentucky Fried Chicken.

McDONALD'S

McDonald's provides diabetic consumers with a card-sized food exchange list for products served in their restaurants. Exchanges are given for each food component separately (bread exchanges for buns, fat exchanges for sauce, meat exchanges for hamburger, and so forth). Here, we have converted those exchanges from high- and medium-fat meat exchanges to lean meat exchanges plus fat, so you can compare the products to others listed. In parentheses, you'll also find the total exchanges for each product as listed on the McDonald's card.

Product Name	Serving Size	Calories	Exchanges
Hamburger	3.6 oz.	260	2 B, 1 M, 1 F (2 B, 1 HF* meat)
Cheeseburger	4.1 oz.	310	2 B, 1½ M, 1½ F (2 B, 1½ HF meat)
Quarter Pounder® sandwich,	5.9 oz.	420	2 B, 2 M, 3 F (2 B, 2 HF meat, 1 F)
with Cheese	6.9 oz.	520	2 B, 3 M, 4 F (2 B, 3 HF meat, 1 F)
Big Mac® sandwich	7.3 oz.	560	2½ B, 2½ M, 5½ F (2½ B, 2½ HF meat, 3 F)
Chicken McNuggets® ***	6 nuggets (4.0 oz.)	310	1 B, 3 M, 2 F (same)
Filet-O-Fish® sandwich	5.0 oz.	430	2½ B, 1½ M, 4 F (2½ B, 1 MF** meat, ½ HF meat, 3 F)
French fries, regular	2.4 oz.	220	2 B, 2 F (same)
Egg McMuffin® sandwich	4.9 oz.	340	2 B, 2 M, 1½ F (2 B, ½ M, 1 MF meat, ½ HF meat)
English muffin,			
Buttered	1 muffin	190	2 B, 1 F (same)
Unbuttered	1 muffin	160	2 B (same)
Hash browns	2.0 oz.	130	1 B, 1 F (same)
Hot cakes,			
with butter, no syrup	7.5 oz.	341	4 B, 1 F (same)
without butter or syrup	7.4 oz.	260	4 B (same)

* HF = high-fat
** MF = medium-fat
*** Sauces for Chicken McNuggets are high in simple sugars and not recommended.

Product Name	Serving Size	Calories	Exchanges
Pork sausage patties	1.9 oz.	210	1 M, 3 F (1 HF meat, 2 F)
Scrambled eggs	3.5 oz.	180	2 M, 2 F (2 MF meat, 1 F)
Juice,			
Grapefruit	6 fl. oz.	80	2 Fr (same)
Orange	6 fl. oz.	80	2 Fr (same)
Milk,			
Low-fat	8 fl. oz.	120	1 F, 1 Mk (same)
Whole	8 fl. oz.	150	2 F, 1 Mk (same)

ROY ROGERS

Product Name	Serving Size	Calories	Exchanges
Hamburger	4 oz.	516	2 B, 3 M, 4½ F
Cheeseburger,	4 oz.	570	2 B, 3½ M, 5 F
Bacon	4 oz.	603	2 B, 4 M, 5½ F
Double-R-Bar burger	4 oz.	672	2½ B, 4½ M, 5½ F
Roast Beef sandwich,	3.25 oz.	459	2½ B, 4½ M, ½ F
with Cheese	3.25 oz.	511	2½ B, 4½ M, 1½ F
Large	4.5 oz.	505	2 B, 6 M, ½ F
with Cheese	4.5 oz.	557	2 B, 6½ M, 1 F
Fried chicken,			
Breasts	8.0 oz.	241	½ B, 2½ M, 1½ F
Drumsticks	4.0 oz.	136	2 M, ½ F
Thighs	6.5 oz.	276	½ B, 2½ M, 2½ F
Wings	3.5 oz.	151	1½ M, 1½ F

Salad Bar and Fixin's Bar

Lettuce, onions, tomato, cucumber, peppers, carrots, radishes, and bean sprouts are free in moderation when used as a garnish for your sandwich. If you use these items in larger amounts, as part of a salad, use standard ADA exchanges for fresh foods. Lettuce, cucumbers, and radishes are free in a salad; one-half cup of onions, tomatoes, carrots, peppers, or bean sprouts equals one vegetable exchange. These may be mixed as desired. Other salad bar items are listed below:

Product Name	Serving Size	Calories	Exchanges
Bacon bits	1 tbsp.	29	½ M
Cheese, Parmesan	1 tsp.	28	½ M
Chick peas	1 oz.	102	1½ B
Chow mein noodles	¼ cup	77	½ B, 1 F

Product Name	Serving Size	Calories	Exchanges
Dressing,			
Blue cheese	2 tbsp.	147	3 F
French	2 tbsp.	116	2½ F
Italian, lo-cal	2 tbsp.	15	free in moderation
Egg, diced	1 tbsp.	23	½ M
Potato salad	¼ cup	74	½ B, 1 F
French fries,			
Regular	3.0 oz.	240	2 B, 2½ F
Large	4.0 oz.	321	2½ B, 3½ F
Juice,			
Apple	6 fl. oz.	56	1½ Fr
Orange	6 fl. oz.	54	1½ Fr
Tomato	6 fl. oz.	29	1 V
Milk, whole	8 fl. oz.	160	1½ F, 1 Mk
Bacon	1 serving	54	1 F
Egg			
Sandwich	1 sandwich	290	2 B, 1½ M, 2 F
Scrambled	1 serving	104	1 M, 1 F
English muffin	2 oz.	130	2 B
Hash browns	1 serving	137	1 B, 1½ F
Ham	1 serving	102	1 M, 1 F
Pancakes	1 serving	229	2½ B, 1 F
Sausage	1 serving	196	1 M, 3 F

TACO BELL

Product Name	Serving Size	Calories	Exchanges
Bellbeefer,	4.4 oz.	221	1½ B, 1½ M, ½ F
with Cheese	4.8 oz.	278	1½ B, 2 M, 1½ F
Burrito,			
Bean	5.9 oz.	343	3 B, 1 M, 2 F
Beef	6.5 oz.	446	2½ B, 3½ M, 2 F
Combination	6.2 oz.	404	3 B, 2 M, 2 F
Supreme	8.0 oz.	457	3 B, 2 M, 3 F
Enchirito	7.3 oz.	454	3 B, 2½ M, 2½ F
Taco,	2.8 oz.	192	1 B, 1 M, 1½ F
Bellgrande	6.5 oz.	410	1½ B, 3 M, 3 F
Light	6.0 oz.	390	1 B, 3 M, 3½ F
Supreme	3.5 oz.	237	1 B, 1½ M, 2 F
Tostada,	5.5 oz.	259	1½ B, 1 M, 2 F
Beefy	6.8 oz.	331	1½ B, 2 M, 2½ F

Product Name	Serving Size	Calories	Exchanges
WENDY'S			
Hamburger,			
Single	7.0 oz.	472	2½ B, 3 M, 3 F
Double	10.0 oz.	669	2½ B, 5 M, 5 F
Triple	12.7 oz.	853	2 B, 9 M, 5 F
Cheeseburger,			
Single	8.5 oz.	577	2½ B, 3½ M, 4½ F
Double	11.5 oz.	797	2½ B, 6½ M, 5½ F
Triple	14.2 oz.	1,035	2½ B, 9½ M, 7½ F
French fries	4.2 oz.	327	2½ B, 3½ F
Chicken sandwich,	7.6 oz.	468	3 B, 3 M, 2 F
with Cheese	8.0 oz.	496	3 B, 2½ M, 3½ F
Chili	8.8 oz.	229	1½ B, 1½ M, 1 F
Taco salad	13.6 oz.	460	2½ B, 3 M, 3 F

10

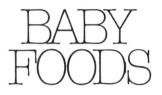

BABY FOODS

☐ Cereals
☐ Strained foods
☐ Junior foods

You may be surprised to find that baby foods are simply adult foods that have been cooked, puréed or strained, and processed. The dry cereal mixes and fruits, juices, meats, vegetables, and combination foods in jars all provide nutrition similar to that of the foods you cook and purée yourself, in convenient portions with standard nutrient levels. Many varieties (except desserts, which are not listed here) are now packaged without added sugar or salt; and many fruits, vegetables, and

juices are enriched with vitamin C. Exchanges for these foods were calculated on the same basis as adult foods. As with all foods, be alert to label information. Many products with the same name have very different formulations, which are reflected in the differing ingredients and ingredient order on the label. We've calculated exchanges to reflect the foods' actual nutrient content as closely as possible.

Once you start looking at these "baby" foods as strained or puréed versions of the foods you eat every day, you'll see they have lots of uses. If you're insulin-dependent and have dental problems that make a soft diet necessary; or if you're ill for a short period and can tolerate only bland, easy-to-digest foods, consider baby foods in your meal plan. They can also be useful for debilitated geriatric patients. And strained fruits and juices provide fast-acting carbohydrate useful for counter-acting insulin reactions.

With the advice and support of your physician and dietitian, baby food exchanges can also be used when planning meals for a diabetic infant. Diabetes is rare in children under two, but is seen occasionally even in newborns. Ninety-eight percent of children with diabetes are insulin-dependent. Planning meals and feeding a diabetic infant requires the closest cooperation of parent, physician, and dietitian. Your physician will help you choose among breast milk, cow's milk, or a soy- or meat-based formula. But as your child makes the transition to other foods, a diet plan must be devised.

An exchange system using prepared baby foods can be a useful approach.* All infants need frequent feedings, but this is even more important for the infant with diabetes, whose food must be distributed throughout the day to balance the insulin dosage. An exchange system can be designed to offer a proper balance and distribution of carbohydrate, protein, fat, vitamins, and minerals throughout the day, which is vital to all infants.

To avoid stress at meals and possible hypoglycemia (low blood sugar), an infant is usually allowed more flexibility in meals than is an adult. Because hypoglycemia can harm an infant's developing brain, slightly higher blood sugars are usually also tolerated. To help ensure both adequate nutrition and good control of blood glucose levels, many parents today combine an exchange-based meal plan with frequent (a minimum of four times a day) monitoring of their diabetic child's blood glucose levels.

We can't make recommendations here about specific meal plans—nutritional requirements vary greatly, and each infant's plan must be individually tailored by the attending physician and dietitian. But a meal plan based on baby food exchanges may make things easier and can teach family members the rudiments of a system they'll use throughout the child's life.

Product Name	Serving Size	Calories	Exchanges
CEREALS			
■ Dry			
Barley,			
Beech-Nut	½ oz.	50	½ B
Gerber	½ oz.	60	1 B
Heinz	½ oz.	50	½ B
High protein,			
Beech-Nut	½ oz.	50	½ B, ½ M
Gerber	½ oz.	50	½ B, ½ M

*Benz, M., and Kohler, E., *Diabetes Care* **3(4):554,** 1980

Product Name	Serving Size	Calories	Exchanges
Heinz	½ oz.	50	½ B, ½ M
with Apple and orange, *Gerber*	½ oz.	60	½ B, ½ M
Mixed,			
Beech-Nut	½ oz.	50	½ B
Gerber	½ oz.	60	1 B
Heinz	½ oz.	60	1 B
with Banana, *Gerber*	½ oz.	60	½ B, ½ Fr
Oatmeal,			
Beech-Nut	½ oz.	50	½ B
Gerber	½ oz.	50	½ B
Heinz	½ oz.	50	½ B
with Banana, *Gerber*	½ oz.	60	½ B, ½ Fr
Rice,			
Beech-Nut	½ oz.	50	½ B
Gerber	½ oz.	60	1 B
Heinz	½ oz.	60	1 B
with Banana, *Gerber*	½ oz.	60	½ B, ½ Fr

■ Jar—Strained

Product Name	Serving Size	Calories	Exchanges
Mixed,			
with Applesauce and bananas,			
Beech-Nut	4½ oz.	80	1 B, ½ Fr
Gerber	4½ oz.	90	1 B, ½ Fr
with Apples and bananas, *Heinz*	4¾ oz.	100	1 B, 1 Fr
Oatmeal with applesauce and bananas,			
Beech-Nut	4½ oz.	90	1 B, ½ Fr
Gerber	4½ oz.	80	1 B, ½ Fr
Heinz	4¾ oz.	100	1 B, 1 Fr
Rice,			
with Applesauce and bananas,			
Beech-Nut	4½ oz.	90	1 B, ½ Fr
Gerber	4¾ oz.	100	1 B, 1 Fr
with Apples and bananas, *Heinz*	4¾ oz.	110	1 B, 1 Fr

■ Jar—Junior

Product Name	Serving Size	Calories	Exchanges
Mixed, with applesauce and bananas, *Gerber*	7½ oz.	140	1½ B, 1 Fr
Oatmeal, with applesauce and bananas, *Gerber*	7½ oz.	130	1½ B, ½ Fr
Rice, with mixed fruit, *Gerber*	7¾ oz.	170	2 B, 1 Fr

Product Name	Serving Size	Calories	Exchanges

STRAINED FOODS

■ Dinners

Beef and egg noodle,

Beech-Nut	4½ oz.	90	1 B, ½ F
Heinz	4½ oz.	60	½ B, ½ F
with Vegetables, *Gerber*	4½ oz.	90	½ B, ½ M, ½ V, ½ F

Beef with vegetables, high meat,

Gerber	4½ oz.	120	½ B, 1 M, ½ F
Heinz	4½ oz.	100	1 M, 1 V, ½ F
and Cereal, *Beech-Nut*	4½ oz.	130	½ B, 1 M, ½ V, ½ F
Cereal and egg yolks, *Gerber*	4½ oz.	70	1 B

Cereal, egg yolks,
and bacon, *Beech-Nut* . . . 4½ oz. . . . 110 . . . 1 B, 1 F

Chicken noodle,

Beech-Nut	4½ oz.	70	1 B
Gerber	4½ oz.	80	1 B
Heinz	4½ oz.	70	½ B, ½ V, ½ F

Chicken rice,

Beech-Nut	4½ oz.	70	1 B

Chicken soup,

Heinz	4½ oz.	70	½ B, ½ V, ½ F
Cream of, *Gerber*	4½ oz.	80	1 B, ½ F

Chicken with vegetables, high meat,

Gerber	4½ oz.	130	½ B, 1 M, ½ V, ½ F
Heinz	4½ oz.	110	1 M, 1 V, ½ F
and Cereal, *Beech-Nut*	4½ oz.	90	½ B, ½ M, ½ V, ½ F
Cottage cheese with pineapple, *Gerber*	4½ oz.	130	1 M, 2 Fr

Ham with vegetables, high meat,

Gerber	4½ oz.	100	½ B, 1 M, ½ V
and Cereal, *Beech-Nut*	4½ oz.	130	½ B, 1 M, ½ V, ½ F
Macaroni and cheese, *Gerber*	4½ oz.	90	½ B, ½ M, ½ F

Macaroni, tomato, and beef,

Beech-Nut	4½ oz.	90	½ B, ½ V, ½ F
Gerber	4½ oz.	80	½ B, ½ V, ½ F
Heinz	4½ oz.	70	½ B, ½ V, ½ F

Turkey rice,

Beech-Nut	4½ oz.	70	1 B
Heinz	4½ oz.	60	½ B, ½ V, ½ F
with Vegetables, *Gerber*	4½ oz.	80	½ B, ½ V, ½ F

Turkey with vegetables, high meat,

Product Name	Serving Size	Calories	Exchanges
Gerber	4½ oz.	130	½ B, 1 M, ½ V, ½ F
Heinz	4½ oz.	120	½ B, ½ M, ½ V, 1 F
Veal with vegetables, high meat,			
Gerber	4½ oz.	80	½ B, ½ M, ½ V
Vegetable bacon,			
Beech-Nut	4½ oz.	90	½ B, ½ V, 1 F
Gerber	4½ oz.	100	½ B, ½ V, 1 F
Heinz	4½ oz.	80	½ B, 1 V, ½ F
Vegetable beef,			
Beech-Nut	4½ oz.	90	½ B, ½ V, 1 F
Gerber	4½ oz.	80	½ B, ½ V, ½ F
Heinz	4½ oz.	70	1 B, ½ M, ½ V
Vegetable chicken,			
Beech-Nut	4½ oz.	80	½ B, ½ V, ½ F
Gerber	4½ oz.	70	½ B, ½ V, ½ F
Vegetables, dumplings, and beef, Heinz	4½ oz.	70	½ B, ½ V, ½ F
Vegetables, egg noodles, and chicken, Heinz	4½ oz.	90	½ B, ½ V, ½ F
Vegetables, egg noodles, and turkey, Heinz	4½ oz.	60	½ B, ½ V, ½ F
Vegetable ham,			
Beech-Nut	4½ oz.	90	½ B, 1 V, ½ F
Gerber	4½ oz.	80	½ B, ½ V, ½ F
Heinz	4½ oz.	60	½ B, 1 V
Vegetables and lamb,			
Gerber	4½ oz.	80	½ B, ½ V, ½ F
with Rice and barley, Beech-Nut	4½ oz.	80	½ B, ½ V, ½ F
Vegetables and liver,			
Gerber	4½ oz.	60	½ B, ½ V
with Rice and barley, Beech-Nut	4½ oz.	70	1 B, ½ V
Vegetable turkey,			
Beech-Nut	4½ oz.	70	½ B, ½ V, ½ F
Gerber	4½ oz.	70	½ B, ½ V, ½ F

■ Fruit

Apples and apricots,			
Beech-Nut	4½ oz.	60	1½ Fr
Heinz	4½ oz.	70	1½ Fr
Apple blueberry, Gerber	4½ oz.	80	2 Fr
Apples and cranberries with tapioca, Heinz	4¾ oz.	90	2 Fr

Product Name	Serving Size	Calories	Exchanges
Apples and nonfat yogurt, *Gerber*	4½ oz.	100	1½ Fr, ½ Mk
Apples and grapes supreme, *Beech-Nut*	4½ oz.	110	2½ Fr
Apples, mandarin oranges, and bananas supreme, *Beech-Nut*	4½ oz.	90	2 Fr
Apples, peaches, and strawberries supreme, *Beech-Nut*	4½ oz.	100	2½ Fr
Apples and pears, *Heinz*	4½ oz.	80	2 Fr
Apples, pears, and bananas supreme, *Beech-Nut*	4½ oz.	100	2½ Fr
Apples, pears, and pineapple supreme, *Beech-Nut*	4½ oz.	100	2½ Fr
Apples and strawberries supreme, *Beech-Nut*	4½ oz.	100	2½ Fr
Applesauce,			
Beech-Nut	4½ oz.	60	1½ Fr
Gerber	4½ oz.	70	1½ Fr
Heinz	4½ oz.	70	1½ Fr
Applesauce and apricots, *Gerber*	4½ oz.	80	2 Fr
Applesauce and bananas, *Beech-Nut*	4½ oz.	60	1½ Fr
Applesauce and cherries, *Beech-Nut*	4½ oz.	70	1½ Fr
Applesauce and raspberries, *Beech-Nut*	4½ oz.	60	1½ Fr
Apricots with tapioca,			
Beech-Nut	4½ oz.	80	2 Fr
Gerber	4¾ oz.	100	2½ Fr
Heinz	4¾ oz.	80	2 Fr
Bananas and nonfat yogurt, *Gerber*	4½ oz.	80	1 Fr, ½ Mk
Bananas and pineapple with tapioca,			
Beech-Nut	4½ oz.	80	2 Fr
Gerber	4½ oz.	70	1½ Fr
Heinz	4¾ oz.	90	2 Fr
Bananas with tapioca,			
Beech-Nut	4½ oz.	80	2 Fr
Gerber	4½ oz.	100	2½ Fr
Heinz	4¾ oz.	110	2½ Fr
Guava, *Gerber*	4½ oz.	90	2 Fr
Guava and papaya, *Gerber*	4½ oz.	90	2 Fr
Island fruits, *Beech-Nut*	4½ oz.	90	2 Fr
Mango, *Gerber*	4¾ oz.	110	2½ Fr
Mango with tapioca, *Beech-Nut*	4½ oz.	90	2 Fr
Mixed fruit and nonfat yogurt, *Gerber*	4½ oz.	110	1½ Fr, ½ Mk

Product Name	Serving Size	Calories	Exchanges
Papaya and applesauce, *Gerber*	4½ oz.	80	2 Fr
Papaya with tapioca, *Beech-Nut*	4½ oz.	80	2 Fr
Peaches,			
Beech-Nut	4½ oz.	90	2 Fr
Gerber	4¾ oz.	100	2½ Fr
Heinz	4½ oz.	50	1 Fr
Pears,			
Beech-Nut	4½ oz.	90	2 Fr
Gerber	4½ oz.	70	1½ Fr
Heinz	4½ oz.	70	1½ Fr
Pears and pineapple, *Beech-Nut*	4½ oz.	100	2½ Fr
Gerber	4½ oz.	80	2 Fr
Heinz	4½ oz.	80	2 Fr
Plums with tapioca,			
Beech-Nut	4½ oz.	90	2 Fr
Gerber	4¾ oz.	100	2½ Fr
Heinz	4½ oz.	80	2 Fr
Prunes with tapioca,			
Beech-Nut	4½ oz.	100	2½ Fr
Gerber	4¾ oz.	110	2½ Fr
Heinz	4¾ oz.	120	3 Fr

■ Juice

Product Name	Serving Size	Calories	Exchanges
Apple,			
Beech-Nut	4¼ fl. oz.	60	1½ Fr
Gerber	4¼ fl. oz.	60	1½ Fr
Heinz	4.2 fl. oz.	60	1½ Fr
Apple-apricot, *Heinz*	4.2 fl. oz.	70	1½ Fr
Apple banana, *Gerber*	4¼ fl. oz.	60	1½ Fr
Apple cherry,			
Beech-Nut	4¼ fl. oz.	50	1 Fr
Gerber	4¼ fl. oz.	60	1½ Fr
Heinz	4.2 fl. oz.	60	1½ Fr
Apple cranberry, *Beech-Nut*	4¼ fl. oz.	60	1½ Fr
Apple grape,			
Beech-Nut	4¼ fl. oz.	60	1½ Fr
Gerber	4¼ fl. oz.	60	1½ Fr
Heinz	4.2 fl. oz.	70	1½ Fr
Apple peach,			
Beech-Nut	4¼ fl. oz.	60	1½ Fr
Gerber	4¼ fl. oz.	60	1½ Fr

Product Name	Serving Size	Calories	Exchanges
Heinz	4.2 oz.	60	1½ Fr
Apple pineapple, *Heinz*	4.2 oz.	60	1½ Fr
Apple plum, *Gerber*	4¼ fl. oz.	60	1½ Fr
Apple prune,			
Beech-Nut	4¼ fl. oz.	70	1½ Fr
Gerber	4¼ fl. oz.	60	1½ Fr
Heinz	4.2 oz.	70	1½ Fr
Mixed,			
Beech-Nut	4¼ fl. oz.	60	1½ Fr
Gerber	4¼ fl. oz.	70	1½ Fr
Heinz	4.2 oz.	70	1½ Fr
Orange,			
Beech-Nut	4¼ fl. oz.	60	1½ Fr
Gerber	4¼ fl. oz.	70	1½ Fr
Heinz	4.2 fl. oz.	60	1½ Fr
Orange apple, *Gerber*	4¼ fl. oz.	70	1½ Fr
Orange-apple-banana, *Heinz*	4.2 fl. oz.	60	1½ Fr
Orange apricot, *Gerber*	4¼ fl. oz.	70	1½ Fr
Orange banana, *Beech-Nut*	4¼ fl. oz.	60	1½ Fr
Orange pineapple, *Gerber*	4¼ fl. oz.	80	2 Fr

■ Meats

Product Name	Serving Size	Calories	Exchanges
Beef and beef broth,			
Beech-Nut	3½ oz.	120	2 M
Heinz	3½ oz.	130	2 M, ½ F
Beef with beef heart and egg yolks, *Gerber*	3.5 oz.	90	2 M
Beef and egg yolk, *Gerber*	3.5 oz.	90	2 M
Beef liver with egg yolks, *Gerber*	3.5 oz.	90	2 M
Chicken and chicken broth,			
Beech-Nut	3½ oz.	110	2 M
Heinz	3½ oz.	130	2 M, ½ F
Chicken with egg yolks, *Gerber*	3.5 oz.	140	2 M, ½ F
Ham with egg yolks, *Gerber*	3.5 oz.	110	2 M
Ham and ham broth, *Beech-Nut*	3½ oz.	120	2 M
Lamb with egg yolks, *Gerber*	3.5 oz.	100	2 M
Lamb with lamb broth,			
Beech-Nut	3½ oz.	130	2 M, ½ F
Heinz	3½ oz.	150	2 M, 1 F
Liver and liver broth, *Heinz*	3½ oz.	90	2 M
Pork with egg yolks, *Gerber*	3.5 oz.	110	2 M

Product Name	Serving Size	Calories	Exchanges
Turkey with egg yolks, *Gerber*	3.5 oz.	120	2 M
Turkey and turkey broth,			
Beech-Nut	3½ oz.	120	2 M
Heinz	3½ oz.	120	2 M
Veal with egg yolks, *Gerber*	3.5 oz.	90	2 M
Veal with veal broth,			
Beech-Nut	3½ oz.	120	2 M
Heinz	3½ oz.	130	2 M, ½ F

■ Vegetables

Product Name	Serving Size	Calories	Exchanges
Beets,			
Beech-Nut	4½ oz.	50	1½ V
Gerber	4½ oz.	50	1½ V
Heinz	4½ oz.	50	1½ V
Carrots,			
Beech-Nut	4½ oz.	40	1½ V
Gerber	4½ oz.	35	1 V
Heinz	4½ oz.	25	1 V
Corn, creamed,			
Beech-Nut	4½ oz.	90	1½ B
Gerber	4½ oz.	90	1½ B
Heinz	4½ oz.	90	1½ B
Garden vegetables,			
Beech-Nut	4½ oz.	60	2 V
Gerber	4½ oz.	50	2 V
Green beans,			
Beech-Nut	4½ oz.	40	1½ V
Gerber	4½ oz.	40	1½ V
Heinz	4½ oz.	40	1½ V
Mixed vegetables,			
Gerber	4½ oz.	60	1 B
Heinz	4½ oz.	60	2 V
Peas,			
Beech-Nut	4½ oz.	70	1 B
Gerber	4½ oz.	60	1 B
Creamed, *Heinz*	4½ oz.	80	1 B, ½ F
Peas and carrots, *Beech-Nut*	4½ oz.	60	½ B, 1 V
Spinach, creamed, *Gerber*	4½ oz.	60	1 V, ½ F
Squash,			
Beech-Nut	4½ oz.	30	½ B
Gerber	4½ oz.	40	½ B

Product Name	Serving Size	Calories	Exchanges
Heinz	4½ oz.	45	½ B
Sweet potatoes,			
Beech-Nut	4½ oz.	70	1 B
Gerber	3¾ oz.	80	1 B
Heinz	4¾ oz.	90	1 B

JUNIOR FOODS

■ Dinners

Product Name	Serving Size	Calories	Exchanges
Beef and egg noodles,			
Beech-Nut	7½ oz.	140	1 B, ½ M, 1 F
with Vegetables, *Gerber*	7½ oz.	140	1 B, ½ M, ½ V, ½ F
Beef with vegetables, high meat,			
Gerber	4½ oz.	130	½ B, 1 M, ½ V, ½ F
and Cereal, *Beech-Nut*	4½ oz.	130	½ B, 1 M, ½ V, ½ F
and Cereal, *Heinz*	4½ oz.	130	1 M, 1 V, 1 F
Cereal and egg yolk, *Gerber*	7½ oz.	110	1 B, 1 F
Chicken noodle,			
Beech-Nut	7½ oz.	120	1 B, 1 F
Gerber	7½ oz.	120	1 B, ½ M, ½ F
Heinz	7½ oz.	150	1 B, 1½ V, 1 F
Chicken with vegetables, high meat,			
Gerber	4½ oz.	130	½ B, 1 M, ½ V, ½ F
Heinz	4½ oz.	120	1 M, 1½ V, ½ F
and Cereal, *Beech-Nut*	4½ oz.	90	½ B, ½ M, ½ V, ½ F
Egg noodles and beef, *Heinz*	7½ oz.	120	1 B, ½ M, 1 V
Ham with vegetables, high meat,			
Gerber	4½ oz.	110	½ B, 1 M, ½ V
and Cereal, *Beech-Nut*	4½ oz.	130	½ B, 1 M, ½ V, ½ F
Macaroni and cheese, *Gerber*	7½ oz.	140	1 B, ½ M, 1 F
Macaroni, tomato, and beef,			
Beech-Nut	7½ oz.	130	1 B, ½ V, 1 F
Gerber	7½ oz.	130	1½ B, ½ V
Heinz	7½ oz.	110	1 B, ½ V, ½ F
Spaghetti, tomato, and beef,			
Beech-Nut	7½ oz.	140	1½ B, ½ V, ½ F
Gerber	7½ oz.	150	1½ B, ½ V, ½ F
Heinz	7½ oz.	130	1 B, ½ M, 1 V
Split peas and ham,			
Beech-Nut	7½ oz.	160	1½ B, ½ M, ½ F
Gerber	7½ oz.	150	1½ B, ½ M, ½ F

Product Name	*Serving Size*	*Calories*	*Exchanges*
Turkey rice, *Beech-Nut*	7½ oz.	130	1½ B, ½ F
Turkey rice with vegetables,			
Gerber	7½ oz.	140	1 B, ½ M, ½ V, ½ F
Heinz	7½ oz.	110	1 B, ½ V, ½ F
Turkey with vegetables, high meat,			
Gerber	4½ oz.	130	½ B, 1 M, ½ V, ½ F
Heinz	4½ oz.	130	½ B, ½ M, 1 V, 1 F
Veal with vegetables, high meat, *Gerber*	4½ oz.	90	½ B, 1 M, ½ V
Vegetable bacon,			
Beech-Nut	7½ oz.	160	1 B, 1 V, 1½ F
Gerber	7½ oz.	170	1 B, 1 V, 1½ F
Heinz	7½ oz.	130	3 V, 1 F
Vegetable beef,			
Beech-Nut	7½ oz.	110	1 B, ½ V, ½ F
Gerber	7½ oz.	140	1 B, ½ M, ½ V, ½ F
Heinz	7½ oz.	120	1 B, ½ M, 1 V
Vegetable chicken,			
Beech-Nut	7½ oz.	130	1 B, ½ M, ½ V, ½ F
Gerber	7½ oz.	110	1 B, ½ V, ½ F
Vegetables, dumplings, and beef, *Heinz*	7½ oz.	110	1 B, 1 V, ½ F
Vegetables, egg noodles, and chicken, *Heinz*	7½ oz.	140	1 B, 1 V, 1 F
Vegetables, egg noodles, and turkey, *Heinz*	7½ oz.	110	1 B, 1 V, 1 F
Vegetables and ham,			
Gerber	7½ oz.	140	1 B, ½ M, ½ V, ½ F
Heinz	7½ oz.	120	1 B, ½ M, 1 V
Vegetables and lamb, *Gerber*	7½ oz.	130	1 B, ½ V, 1 F
Vegetable lamb with rice and barley, *Beech-Nut*	7½ oz.	130	1 B, ½ V, 1 F
Vegetables and liver, *Gerber*	7½ oz.	90	1 B, ½ V
Vegetable liver with rice and barley, *Beech-Nut*	7½ oz.	120	1 B, ½ M, ½ V

■ Fruits

Apples and apricots,			
Beech-Nut	7½ oz.	90	2 Fr
Heinz	7½ oz.	110	2½ Fr
Apple blueberry, *Gerber*	7½ oz.	120	3 Fr
Apples and cranberries with tapioca, *Heinz*	7¾ oz.	140	3½ Fr

Product Name	Serving Size	Calories	Exchanges
Apples and grapes supreme, *Beech-Nut*	7½ oz.	190	4½ Fr
Apples, mandarin oranges, and bananas supreme, *Beech-Nut*	7½ oz.	150	3½ Fr
Apples, peaches, and strawberries supreme, *Beech-Nut*	7½ oz.	160	4 Fr
Apples and pears, *Heinz*	7¾ oz.	130	3 Fr
Apples, pears, and bananas supreme, *Beech-Nut*	7½ oz.	160	4 Fr
Apples, pears, and pineapples supreme, *Beech-Nut*	7½ oz.	160	4 Fr
Apples and strawberries supreme, *Beech-Nut*	7½ oz.	160	4 Fr
Applesauce,			
Beech-Nut	7½ oz.	100	2½ Fr
Gerber	7½ oz.	110	2½ Fr
Heinz	7½ oz.	110	2½ Fr
Applesauce and apricots, *Gerber*	7½ oz.	110	2½ Fr
Applesauce and bananas, *Beech-Nut*	7½ oz.	110	2½ Fr
Applesauce and cherries, *Beech-Nut*	7½ oz.	110	2½ Fr
Applesauce and raspberries, *Beech-Nut*	7½ oz.	100	2½ Fr
Apricots with tapioca,			
Beech-Nut	7½ oz.	140	3½ Fr
Gerber	7¾ oz.	160	4 Fr
Heinz	7¾ oz.	150	3½ Fr
Bananas and pineapple with tapioca,			
Beech-Nut	7½ oz.	120	3 Fr
Gerber	7½ oz.	120	3 Fr
Heinz	7¾ oz.	150	3½ Fr
Bananas with tapioca,			
Beech-Nut	7½ oz.	130	3 Fr
Gerber	7½ oz.	150	3½ Fr
Heinz	7¾ oz.	180	4 Fr, ½ F
Guava with tapioca, *Beech-Nut*	7½ oz.	140	3½ Fr
Island fruit, *Beech-Nut*	7½ oz.	150	3½ Fr
Mango with tapioca, *Beech-Nut*	7½ oz.	150	3½ Fr
Papaya with tapioca, *Beech-Nut*	7½ oz.	140	3½ Fr
Peaches,			
Beech-Nut	7½ oz.	150	3½ Fr
Gerber	7¾ oz.	160	4 Fr
Heinz	7¾ oz.	90	2 Fr

Product Name	Serving Size	Calories	Exchanges
Pears,			
Beech-Nut	7½ oz.	140	3½ Fr
Gerber	7½ oz.	120	3 Fr
Heinz	7½ oz.	120	3 Fr
Pears and pineapple,			
Beech-Nut	7½ oz.	160	4 Fr
Gerber	7½ oz.	120	3 Fr
Plums with tapioca,			
Beech-Nut	7½ oz.	150	3½ Fr
Gerber	7¾ oz.	170	4 Fr
Prunes with tapioca, *Gerber*	7¾ oz.	180	4½ Fr

■ Meats

Product Name	Serving Size	Calories	Exchanges
Beef, *Gerber*	3½ oz.	100	2 M
Beef and beef broth,			
Beech-Nut	3½ oz.	130	2 M, ½ F
Heinz	3½ oz.	130	2 M, ½ F
Chicken, *Gerber*	3½ oz.	140	2 M, ½ F
Chicken and chicken broth,			
Beech-Nut	3½ oz.	110	2 M
Heinz	3½ oz.	130	2 M, ½ F
Chicken sticks, *Gerber*	2½ oz.	120	1½ M, 1 F
Ham, *Gerber*	3½ oz.	120	2 M
Lamb, *Gerber*	3½ oz.	100	2 M
Lamb and lamb broth,			
Beech-Nut	3½ oz.	130	2 M, ½ F
Heinz	3½ oz.	150	2 M, 1 F
Meat sticks, *Gerber*	2½ oz.	110	1½ M, ½ F
Turkey, *Gerber*	3½ oz.	130	2 M, ½ F
Turkey sticks, *Gerber*	2½ oz.	120	1½ M, 1 F
Veal, *Gerber*	3½ oz.	100	2 M
Veal and veal broth, *Heinz*	3½ oz.	130	2 M, ½ F

■ Vegetables

Product Name	Serving Size	Calories	Exchanges
Carrots,			
Beech-Nut	7½ oz.	60	2 V
Gerber	7½ oz.	60	2 V
Heinz	7½ oz.	55	2 V
Corn, creamed,			
Beech-Nut	7½ oz.	150	2 B
Gerber	7½ oz.	130	2 B

Product Name	Serving Size	Calories	Exchanges
Heinz	7¾ oz.	160	2 B, ½ F
Green beans,			
Beech-Nut	7¼ oz.	60	2 V
Creamed, *Heinz*	7½ oz.	90	2 V, 1 F
Mixed vegetables,			
Beech-Nut	7½ oz.	80	1 B
Gerber	7½ oz.	90	1½ B
Peas,			
Beech-Nut	7½ oz.	110	1½ B
Gerber	7½ oz.	140	2 B
Creamed, *Heinz*	7½ oz.	140	1 B, 1 F
Squash,			
Beech-Nut	7½ oz.	50	1 B
Gerber	7½ oz.	70	1 B
Sweet potatoes,			
Beech-Nut	7½ oz.	120	1½ B
Gerber	7¾ oz.	140	2 B
Heinz	7½ oz.	140	2 B

11

ALCOHOLIC BEVERAGES

☐ Beer
☐ Wine
☐ Distilled spirits

Alcohol use, once considered taboo for diabetics, has been reconsidered in recent years. The American Diabetes Association Committee on Food and Nutrition now states that, "With the approval of the responsible physician, alcoholic beverages in prescribed amounts may be consumed by diabetic persons."* However, you should observe certain precautions.

Alcohol should be consumed only if your diabetes is well-controlled, and only with your physician's knowledge. Because it can produce a hypoglycemic reaction (low blood sugar), alcohol should be consumed only with food, preferably with a meal (or shortly before or after one). Insulin-dependent diabetics should be particularly careful to avoid situations where cocktails are served before a dinner party that's scheduled much later than their normal mealtime. The combined hypoglycemic effects of a few drinks and a delayed mealtime can be disastrous, especially since symptoms of hypoglycemia may resemble those of intoxication. Proper treatment for you may be delayed because those around you

---

* *Diabetes Care* 2(6):520,1979

will assume you have simply overindulged.

Because alcohol may stimulate your appetite, beware of the "munchie effect." You may find yourself sorely tempted by displays of *hors d'oeuvre* or an overly generous dinner. Those extra calories, plus the calories provided by the alcohol itself, can wreak havoc with your diet.

In some people, alcohol also interacts with certain oral hypoglycemic agents (blood-sugar-lowering pills) to produce hot flashes, dizziness, headache, nausea, and breathlessness—a group of symptoms known as a "disulfiram-like reaction." If you are taking an oral hypoglycemic, be sure to talk with your physician before consuming any alcoholic beverages.

The amount of alcohol you can safely drink depends upon your weight and how well your diabetes is controlled, and should be discussed with your physician. Recommendations will vary, but in general you should drink no more than two glasses of wine, two cans of beer, or two jiggers of distilled spirits per day.

Once you know how much you can drink, you then need to know *what* you can drink. Sweet dessert and appetizer wines (up to 15% sugar), cordials or liqueurs (up to 50% sugar), sweetened mixed drinks, and mixed drinks made with sugar-sweetened beverages should be considered off-limits because of their high sugar content. Beer and ale contain significant amounts of carbohydrate, which you must take into account in your meal plan. Distilled spirits (brandy, gin, rum, tequila, vodka, and whiskey) contain no carbohydrate. Dry red, white, and rosé table wines, dry champagne, dry sherry, and dry vermouth have very small amounts of carbohydrate that you can safely disregard.

Non-insulin-dependent diabetics who are on weight-control diets should count the calories from alcohol in their meal plan. Because the body metabolizes it like fat, alcohol is commonly worked into the meal plan as fat exchanges, which are subtracted from the total allowed for your meal. However, you may also use bread exchanges to account for the calories in alcohol, if this is more convenient.

Insulin-dependent diabetics should not substitute alcoholic beverages for other exchanges. The American Diabetes Association suggests that insulin-dependent diabetics at ideal body weight simply count the alcohol as extra calories in addition to their regular meal plan.* Because of the possibility of alcohol-induced hypoglycemia, you should make sure to eat all your regular exchanges.

If you use alcohol in combination with a caloric mixer such as orange juice, tomato juice, or cream, remember to count the appropriate number of fruit, vegetable, or fat exchanges (see Chapters 3 and 4). Wine used in moderate amounts for cooking (1 to 2 tablespoons per serving) does not have to be counted in your meal plan, because the alcohol and its calories evaporate during cooking, leaving only the flavor behind.

Listed below are the average number of calories, fat exchange equivalents, and bread exchange equivalents for common alcoholic beverages, so you can work them into your meal plan however you, your physician, and your dietitian find most appropriate. A fat exchange is equivalent to 45 calories; a bread exchange is equivalent to 68 calories. Distilled spirits are listed by proof (a measure of alcohol percentage) rather than name or type, because all spirits of a given proof have the same number of calories.

A Guide for Professionals: The Effective Application of "Exchange Lists for Meal Planning." American Diabetes Association, Inc., and The American Dietetic Association, New York, 1977.

BEER

Because of the high carbohydrate content of beer (approximately 13 grams per 12-ounce serving for regular beer, and 3 to 6 grams per 12-ounce serving for light beer), some bread exchanges should be counted even if you are calculating the alcohol in beer as fat exchanges. Items marked with a • are very low in carbohydrate (3 grams or less), and can be counted solely as fat exchanges.

Product	Serving Size	Calories	Bread Exchanges	Fat Exchanges
Andekar	12 oz. (1 can)	160	2½	or.. 2, + 1 bread
Budweiser	"	144	2	or.. 1½, + 1 bread
Budweiser Light	"	110	1½	or.. 1½, + 1 bread
Busch	"	146	2	or.. 1½, + 1 bread
Hamm's	"	140	2	or.. 1½, + 1 bread
•Hamm's Special Light	"	99	1½	or...... 2
•Jacob Best Premium Light	"	96	1½	or...... 2
Michelob	"	161	2½	or.. 2, + 1 bread
Michelob Light	"	132	2	or.. 1½, + 1 bread
Miller High Life	"	150	2	or.. 2, + 1 bread
•Miller Lite	"	96	1½	or...... 2
Natural Light	"	110	1½	or. 1½, + ½ bread
Old English "800"	"	155	2½	or. 2½, + ½ bread
Olympia	"	150	2	or.. 2, + 1 bread
•Olympia Gold	"	70	1	or...... 1½
Pabst Blue Ribbon	"	150	2	or.. 2, + 1 bread
Pabst Extra Light	"	70	1	or.. 1, + ½ bread

WINE

■ Appetizer

	Serving Size	Calories	Bread Exchanges	Fat Exchanges
Dry port	2 oz. (sherry glass)	80	1	or...... 2
Dry sherry	"	70	1	or...... 1½
Dry vermouth	"	68	1	or...... 1½

■ Table Wines

Dry champagne and dry reds, whites, and rosés containing less than 1% sugar (or 1 gram per 3½-ounce serving) are acceptable. Listed below are a number of varieties low in sugar. Values shown are for *Inglenook* wines; other brands of the same varieties will have similar exchanges.

Product	Serving Size	Calories	Bread Exchanges	Fat Exchanges
Burgundy	3½ oz. (wine glass)	72	1	or 1½
Cabernet Rosé	"	78	1	or 1½
Cabernet Sauvignon	"	77	1	or 1½
Chablis	"	71	1	or 1½
Chardonnay	"	79	1	or 1½
Chenin Blanc	"	75	1	or 1½
Fumé Blanc	"	74	1	or 1½
Gamay Beaujolais	"	74	1	or 1½
Gamay Rosé	"	71	1	or 1½
Gewürztraminer	"	74	1	or 1½
Grey Riesling	"	73	1	or 1½
Johannisberg Riesling	"	74	1	or 1½
Petite Sirah	"	74	1	or 1½
Pinot Chardonnay	"	77	1	or 1½
Pinot Noir	"	77	1	or 1½
Zinfandel	"	77	1	or 1½

DISTILLED SPIRITS (Brandy, gin, rum, tequila, vodka, whiskey)

Values are the same for all brands. The number of calories (and exchanges) depends on the "proof," or alcohol content, of the beverage.

Product	Serving Size	Calories	Bread Exchanges	Fat Exchanges
80 proof	1½ oz. (1 jigger)	97	1½	or 2
84 proof	"	103	1½	or 2½
86 proof	"	105	1½	or 2½
90 proof	"	110	1½	or 2½
94 proof	"	116	1½	or 2½
97 proof	"	121	2	or 3
100 proof	"	124	2	or 3

Appendix I

EQUIVALENTS AND CONVERSIONS

EQUIVALENTS

Volume

3 teaspoons   = 1 tablespoon
2 tablespoons = 1 fluid ounce
8 fluid ounces = 1 cup
16 fluid ounces = 2 cups = 1 pint
32 fluid ounces = 4 cups = 2 pints = 1 quart
64 fluid ounces = 8 cups = 4 pints = 2 quarts = ½ gallon
128 fluid ounces = 16 cups = 8 pints = 4 quarts = 1 gallon

Weight

16 ounces   = 1 pound

CONVERSIONS

Volume

1 teaspoon   =   5 milliliters
1 tablespoon   = 15 milliliters
1 fluid ounce   = 30 milliliters
1 cup   = 240 milliliters (about ¼ liter)
1 pint   = 480 milliliters (about ½ liter)
1 quart   = 960 milliliters (about 1 liter)

Weight

1 ounce   = 28 grams
1 pound   = 454 grams (about ½ kilogram)

Appendix II

FREE AND FREE-IN-MODERATION FOODS

Free foods have few or no calories and can be used in your meal plan as often as you like. Included in this list are beverages, condiments, spices, and seasonings, all of which can add color, interest, and texture to your meals.

Free-in-moderation foods have fewer than 20 calories per serving, not enough to be counted as an exchange. However, they should not be used indiscriminately. If you stick to the amounts suggested, these foods will enhance your meals while adding only a few calories. But if the total amount you eat exceeds 50 calories, you should talk to your dietitian about adjusting your daily exchanges. You may also want to restrict your intake of saccharin-sweetened foods.

Free and free-in-moderation foods are listed here by generic names, to help you with meal planning. Check listings in the appropriate chapters for specific brand names to find serving sizes and an exact calorie count for free-in-moderation foods.

FREE FOODS

Carbonated beverages, sugar-free*
Chewing gum, sugar-free*
Club soda, seltzer, mineral water
Coffee, instant or regular
Flavoring extracts (almond, anise, vanilla, etc.)
Herbs
Herbal teas
Horseradish
Hot sauce
Iced tea mix, unsweetened or sugar-free*

Lemon juice
Lime juice
Nonstick pan spray
Seasoned salts
Soft drink mixes, unsweetened or sugar-free*
Spices
Table-top sweeteners (4 calories per packet or teaspoon, or less)
Tea
Vinegar

*Sweetened with saccharin or aspartame (**NutraSweet**). Items sweetened with fructose or sorbitol are *not* free.

FREE-IN-MODERATION FOODS

"Bacon" chips, imitation
Bamboo shoots
Bean sprouts
Bouillon, fat-free
Broth
Catsup
Cereal beverages
Chile peppers
Chile salsa
Chili sauce
Cocktail sauce
Consommé
Cooking wine
Creamers, nondairy
Croutons

Enchilada sauce
Gelatin, unsweetened or sugar-free
Gravy flavorings and mixes
Hard candy, sugar-free
Jams and jellies, dietetic
Meat marinade mix
Mustard
Pickles, unsweetened
Relish, unsweetened
Salad dressing, low-calorie
Soy sauce
Steak sauce
Taco sauce
Whipped topping mix, reduced-calorie
Worcestershire sauce

Appendix III

FOODS FOR SICK DAYS

Because seemingly minor illnesses such as flu, colds, upset stomach, and diarrhea may cut down your appetite, they can pose problems for the insulin-dependent diabetic. Major dental work can have the same effect. But you *must* take your insulin; your body needs it just as much as when you are healthy. If your physician gives you special rules for the amount of insulin to take during a short-term illness, you should follow these rules without any changes.

If you can't eat your normal meals, however, you must eat the amount of carbohydrate equivalent to your exchanges in order to balance your prescribed amount of insulin. If you can't tolerate meat and fat, you can ignore those exchanges for a few meals during a short-term illness (1 to 3 days). But bread exchanges, fruit exchanges, vegetable exchanges, and milk exchanges all provide carbohydrate and must be replaced.

When ill, you may find liquids and soft foods easier to tolerate than solids, and they'll also help prevent dehydration. During a short illness, regular soft drinks, ice cream, sherbet, popsicles, custard, gelatin, pudding, tapioca, and fruited yogurts that you would normally avoid may be permitted, because they provide concentrated amounts of carbohydrate.

If you are feeling up to it, you can just eat your normal bread, fruit, milk, and vegetable exchanges. If not, you can easily figure out the amount of carbohydrate to replace for each meal by translating all your exchanges into "bread exchanges" (15 grams of carbohydrate), which you can then replace with easy-to-digest foods. (Do this figuring for each meal *before* you get sick. Tape a copy of the list inside your medicine cabinet or bedside table—then you won't have to fuss with it when you don't feel well. If you have problems, ask your dietitian for help.)

Here's how to make your list:

1. List the amount of bread, milk, fruit, and vegetable exchanges in your meal. Your breakfast meal plan might look like this:

Bread exchanges:	2	
Milk exchanges:	1	(Ignore your meat and
Fruit exchanges:	1	fat exchanges)
Vegetable exchanges:	0	

2. Now, list the grams of carbohydrate in one exchange:

Bread exchange:	15 grams carbohydrate
Milk exchange:	12 grams carbohydrate
Fruit exchange:	10 grams carbohydrate
Vegetable exchange:	5 grams carbohydrate

3. Multiply the number of exchanges in each category by the number of grams of carbohydrate, and add up the total amount of carbohydrate for your meal:

Bread exchanges:	2 exchanges × 15 grams	30 grams
Milk exchanges:	1 exchange × 12 grams	12 grams
Fruit exchanges:	1 exchange × 10 grams	10 grams
Vegetable exchanges:	0 exchanges × 5 grams	0 grams
	Total Carbohydrate:	52 grams

4. Find the total number of "bread exchanges" for your meal by dividing the total number of carbohydrates (see **Step #3**) by 15 (the number of grams of carbohydrate in a bread exchange).

52 grams of carbohydrate ÷ 15 grams per bread exchange
= 3½ "bread exchanges"

(Round off your figure to the nearest one-half bread exchange.)

Now that you know how many "bread exchanges" will replace the total carbohydrate in your meal, here are some simple, easy-to-digest foods that are high in carbohydrate, and their equivalents in "bread exchanges":

Cereals (oatmeal, Cream of Wheat,
Cream of Rice) . . . . ½ cup . . . . 1 B

Crackers,

Animal crackers . . . . 15 crackers . . . . . 1 B

Saltines . . . . 7 crackers . . . . . 1 B

Cream soups (cream of mushroom,
cream of celery, etc.) . . . . 1 cup . . . . 1 B

Custard . . . . ½ cup . . . . 1 B

Gelatin (*not* artificially sweetened) . . . . ½ cup . . . . . 1½ B

Honey . . . . 1 tbsp. . . . . 1 B

Ice cream . . . . ½ cup . . . . 1 B

Ice milk . . . . ½ cup . . . . 1 B

Juice,

Apple . . . . 4 oz. . . . . 1 B

Cranberry . . . . 3 oz. . . . . 1 B

Grape . . . . 3 oz. . . . . 1 B

Orange . . . . 4 oz. . . . . 1 B

Popsicles . . . . 1 popsicle . . . . . 1 B
Pudding . . . . 3 oz. . . . . . 1½ B
Soft drinks (*not* artificially sweetened) . . . . 4 oz. . . . . 1 B
Sugar . . . . 2 tsp. . . . . . . ½ B
Yogurt,
    Plain . . . . 1 cup . . . . 1 B
    Flavored (coffee, lemon, vanilla) . . . . 1 cup . . . . 2 B
    Fruited . . . . 1 cup . . . . 3 B

If there are other foods you tolerate well when you are sick, look them up in the main part of this book and add them, with their "bread exchanges," to your sick-day list. In terms of carbohydrate content, one milk exchange is roughly equal to one bread exchange; one fruit exchange is equal to two-thirds of a bread exchange; and one vegetable exchange is equal to one-third of a bread exchange.

Also remember that, although they don't replace carbohydrate, broths and bouillons are helpful when you are sick, replacing fluids and necessary minerals. Milk-based foods such as cream soup and yogurt provide some protein and fat as well as carbohydrate.

Using this list, suggestions for replacing the carbohydrate in the sample breakfast shown here might be:

—1½ cups (12 oz., or 1 can) of ginger ale (3 bread exchanges) and 8 animal crackers (½ bread exchange)
—1 cup of ice cream (2 bread exchanges) and ¾ cup (6 oz.) of ginger ale (1½ bread exchanges)
—14 saltines (2 bread exchanges) and ¾ cup (6 oz.) of apple juice (1½ bread exchanges)
—1 cup of lemon-flavored yogurt (2 bread exchanges) and ¾ cup (6 oz.) of ginger ale (1½ bread exchanges)
—1 cup Cream of Wheat (2 bread

exchanges) and 4½ oz. of cranberry juice (1½ bread exchanges)
—18 saltines (2½ bread exchanges) and a cup of tea with a tablespoon of honey (1 bread exchange).

When you make your list of the bread exchanges you need to replace for each sick-day meal, you may also want to write down some sample "menus" of foods that appeal to you when you are sick. But remember:

•Use these rules only during *short-term illnesses* and only for a few meals at a time.

•Take the amount of insulin recommended by your physician for use during illness.

•Test your urine for ketones and sugar at frequent intervals, as recommended by your physician.

•Rest, keep warm, and drink plenty of fluids.

•Call your physician if your illness lasts longer than 48 hours (when you call, have the results of your urine sugar and ketone tests available). Also, call him or her any time you are vomiting or having diarrhea, or if you can't eat the foods on your regular meal plan for more than three or four meals. In addition to the items on this list, your physician may recommend special foods to replace the protein, fat, vitamins, and minerals you are missing.

Appendix IV

AGENCIES, ORGANIZATIONS, AND PUBLICATIONS FOR FURTHER INFORMATION

American Association of Diabetes Educators
North Woodbury Road
Box 56
Pitman, NJ 08071
(609) 589-4831

Promotes diabetes education, supports research, and provides guidance in establishing local chapters of diabetes educators. Their journal, *The Diabetes Educator*, is published quarterly.

American Diabetes Association
2 Park Avenue
New York, NY 10016
(212) 683-7444

Association of physicians, health professionals, and lay people, with affiliate organizations across the country. Their goals are to promote the search for a cure for diabetes and to improve the health and well-being of people with diabetes and their families. They distribute information to the public, offer a wide variety of patient education and family services, and can provide the names of diabetes specialists in your area. *Exchange Lists for Meal Planning* is available through local ADA affiliates. *Diabetes Forecast*, a magazine for diabetics and their families, is published bimonthly; a one-year

subscription is $15. *Diabetes '84*, a quarterly patient newsletter, is free. The ADA also publishes *Diabetes Care*, a bimonthly journal for health professionals.

The American Dietetic Association
430 North Michigan Avenue
Chicago, IL 60611
(312) 280-5000

Professional organization of dietitians that sets standards for education and experience. They can provide lists of qualified dietitians in your area.

Canadian Diabetes Association
78 Bond Street
Toronto, Ontario
M5B 2J8
Canada
(416) 362-4440

In Canada, diabetics employ a Food Group System, which uses "Choices" rather than exchanges to simplify meal planning. The CDA's leaflet, "Good Health Eating Guide," is free for the asking. The National Office can also direct you to local branches.

Diabetes in the News
P.O. Box 3105
Elkhart, IN 46515

Tabloid newsletter published by Ames

Education Corporation. Stories include up-to-date information on diabetes management, diet, and recipes. A one-year (six-issue) subscription costs $6.00.

Juvenile Diabetes Foundation International
23 East 26th Street
New York, NY 10010
(212) 889-7575

Organization of juvenile diabetics and their families that provides counseling and support services. They publish brochures and pamphlets and distribute films and other educational materials.

National Diabetes Information
 Clearinghouse
P.O. Box NDIC
Bethesda, MD 20205
(301) 496-7433 or (202) 842-7630

The NDIC responds to all requests for information about diabetes. They can provide information about available health-care supplies and instruments, statistics on diabetes, teaching manuals, bibliographies, and the names and addresses of diabetes organizations and professional groups in your area. Publications include *Diabetes Dateline*, a bimonthly newsletter for health professionals; *Resource Directory*, a list of state and federal programs offering services and financial assistance to people with diabetes; and topical bibliographies that provide full ordering and price information, such as *Cookbooks for People with Diabetes* and *Sports and Exercise for People with Diabetes.*

Sugarfree Center, Inc.
P.O. Box 114
Van Nuys, California 91408
(213) 994-1093

Mail-order source for diabetes self-care products, books, and information. Write for a free copy of their newsletter, *Health-O-Gram.*

Don't forget to check your local resources. Hospitals in your area may offer diabetes clinics and diabetes teaching sessions. Chapters of The American Dietetic Association in many large cities offer a "Dial-A-Dietitian" service that can provide quick answers to diet and nutrition questions. Local chapters of the American Diabetes Association and the Juvenile Diabetes Foundation can help you solve all kinds of problems.

Appendix V

CALCULATING EXCHANGES FOR OTHER BRAND-NAME FOODS

For brand-name foods not listed here, you can figure out your own exchanges from the list of ingredients and the nutrition information on the label. Manufacturers of over half the packaged foods available now provide nutrition labels—either voluntarily or because of an FDA regulation that requires this labeling for any food to which a nutrient is added or for which a nutrition claim (such as "dietetic" or "low-sodium") is made. If the product you are interested in doesn't carry a nutrition label, write the manufacturer for the grams of carbohydrate, protein, and fat per serving. Without this information, you won't be able to calculate the exchanges.

The portion of the label that you'll be interested in looks like this:

Corned Beef Hash	
Serving Size:	7½ oz.
Servings per Container:	2
Calories:	410
Protein:	17 grams
Carbohydrate:	17 grams
Fat:	30 grams
Sodium:	1.42 g (1420 mg)

Also look at the ingredients list:
Beef and cooked corned beef, rehydrated potatoes, water, salt, spice, sodium nitrate, gum arabic, natural onion flavoring.

The first ingredient listed is present in the largest amount (by weight), the second ingredient listed is present in the second-largest amount, and so forth.

Now, how do you translate all of this information into exchanges? Look at the nutrition label and:

1. *List* the major ingredients:
    Beef and cooked corned beef
    Potatoes

2. *Determine* into which exchange lists the major ingredients fall, using the table in the front of this book:
    Beef and cooked corned beef = meat and fat (or high-fat meat)
    Potatoes = bread

3. *Look up* the values for the exchanges you are using in the table:

Meat = 0 g carbohydrate, 7 g protein, 3 g fat, 55 calories
Fat = 0 g carbohydrate, 0 g protein, 5 g fat, 45 calories
Bread = 15 g carbohydrate, 2 g protein, 0 g fat, 68 calories*

Now, take a deep breath, reach for your pocket calculator, and:

4. *List* the grams of carbohydrate, protein, and fat found on the nutrition label in three columns:

Carbohydrate	Protein	Fat
17	17	30

5. *Subtract* the number of grams of the exchanges you determined in **Step #3**. Start with the exchange for the first ingredient, then move on to the rest. If the number of grams in a column is double or triple the number in the exchange, subtract two or three times the value of the exchange:

	Carbohydrate	Protein	Fat
Values from nutrition label	17	17	30
Subtract 2 meats (beef)	− 0	−14 (7×2)	− 6 (3×2)
remainder:	17	3	24
Subtract 4 fats (beef)	− 0	− 0	−20 (5×4)
remainder:	17	3	4
Subtract 1 bread (potatoes)	−15	− 2	− 0
remainder:	2	1	4

6. *Check* to see how close your exchanges are to the actual calories, by adding up the calories for the exchanges you've determined:

1 bread	= 68 calories
2 meats	= 110 calories (55×2)
4 fats	= 180 calories (45×4)
Total:	358 calories
	(Reported calories equal 410)

You should be within 20 calories of the figure on the label. If not, you need to do some further calculating.

7. *Examine* the grams of carbohydrate, protein, and fat left as your remainder after the subtractions in **Step #5**, and see to which exchange group the remainder most closely corresponds. (Remember

---

*The exact value of a bread exchange is 68 calories. If it's more convenient, you can use the rounded-off figure of 70, as listed in the table.

to consider half exchanges.) In this case, 2 grams of carbohydrate, 1 gram of protein, and 4 grams of fat correspond most closely to 1 fat exchange (0 g carbohydrate, 0 g protein, 5 g fat, 45 calories).

   8. *Add* the calories for the exchange determined for the remainder to your original total from **Step #6.**

$$
\begin{array}{ll}
358 \text{ calories} & \text{(1 bread, 2 meats, 4 fats)} \\
+\ \ 45 \text{ calories} & \text{(1 fat)} \\
\hline
403 \text{ calories} & \text{(Total exchanges:} \\
& \text{1 bread, 2 meats, 5 fats)}
\end{array}
$$

You should now be close in both calories and carbohydrate, protein, and fat content.

   Use the same procedure for products containing milk, fruit, or vegetable exchanges, substituting the appropriate values. With practice, you'll get faster at calculating exchanges. If you feel confused by the procedure, try a few and then have your dietitian go over the results with you before you work these foods into your meal plan.

Appendix VI

SAMPLE EXCHANGE PATTERNS*

The exchange patterns shown below offer only one example for each calorie level. (The particular calorie level right for you is determined by your size and your need to lose, gain, or maintain weight.) Many variations in the patterns that maintain the balance of 50% of calories from carbohydrate, 20% from protein, and 30% from fat are possible. If, for example, you don't drink three servings of milk per day, your dietitian might reduce your milk exchanges and increase your

bread and meat exchanges to achieve the same carbohydrate and protein levels. Vegetable exchanges can be increased or decreased with a corresponding decrease or increase in other exchanges.

But don't attempt to change the patterns yourself, as you'll upset the careful balance of carbohydrate, protein, and fat. Ask your dietitian for help in choosing an exchange pattern at an appropriate calorie level that takes your eating habits into account.

	1000 calories	1200 calories	1300 calories	1400 calories	1500 calories	1600 calories	1700 calories	1800 calories	1900 calories	2000 calories
Skim Milk	2	2	3	3	3	3	3	3	3	3
Vegetable	2	3	3	4	4	4	4	4	4	4
Fruit	3	4	4	4	4	5	5	6	6	6
Bread	4	5	5	5	6	6	7	7	8	9
Lean Meat	4	4	4	5	5	5	6	7	7	7
Fat	4	5	5	6	7	8	8	8	8	9

*Exchange patterns courtesy of Barbara Herbst, M.S., R.D.

INDEX